Underbelly

Childhood Diarrhea and the Hidden Local Realities of Global Health

Rachel Hall-Clifford

foreword by Waleska López Canu
afterword by Arthur Kleinman

The MIT Press
Cambridge, Massachusetts
London, England

The MIT Press would like to thank the anonymous peer reviewers who provided comments on drafts of this book. The generous work of academic experts is essential for establishing the authority and quality of our publications. We acknowledge with gratitude the contributions of these otherwise uncredited readers.

This book was set in Stone Serif and Stone Sans by Westchester Publishing Services. Printed and bound in the United States of America.

Library of Congress Cataloging-in-Publication Data

Names: Hall-Clifford, Rachel, author. | López Canu, Waleska, writer of foreword. | Kleinman, Arthur, writer of afterword.
Title: Underbelly : childhood diarrhea and the hidden local realities of global health / Rachel Hall-Clifford; foreword by Waleska López Canu; afterword by Arthur Kleinman.
Description: Cambridge, Massachusetts : The MIT Press, [2024] | Includes bibliographical references and index.
Identifiers: LCCN 2023024694 (print) | LCCN 2023024695 (ebook) | ISBN 9780262547765 (paperback) | ISBN 9780262378291 (epub) | ISBN 9780262378284 (pdf)
Subjects: MESH: Access to Primary Care | Diarrhea—prevention & control | Fluid Therapy—economics | Global Health—economics | Program Evaluation | Socioeconomic Disparities in Health | Guatemala
Classification: LCC RJ456.D5 (print) | LCC RJ456.D5 (ebook) | NLM W 67 DG5 | DDC 618.92/3427—dc23/eng/20231006
LC record available at https://lccn.loc.gov/2023024694
LC ebook record available at https://lccn.loc.gov/2023024695

10 9 8 7 6 5 4 3 2 1

Underbelly

For
F
and
everyone who still believes
a better world is possible.

Contents

List of Figures and Tables

Figures

Tables

Acknowledgments

This book started with my dissertation work, which was supported by Boston University and the Whiting Foundation. My generous graduate school advisers and committee members shaped my thinking about my data, questioned my assumptions, and encouraged me: Kris Heggenhougen, Jean Jackson, Fredrik Barth, Robert LeVine, Sarah Richards, Charles Lindholm, and Richard Cash. I am forever indebted to Robert Weller and the MGW for clearheaded advice and support. Thank you to Celeste Ray, Elisabeth Hsu, and Stanley Ulijaszek for making me an anthropologist, and to Arthur Kleinman, David Addiss, Jim Lavery, Bob Cook-Deegan, Doug Falen, Martha Rees, and Michelle Lampl for making me want to stay one.

Ongoing work and further research in the Guatemalan health sector have been supported by the US National Institutes of Health and the National Association for the Practice of Anthropology-Occupational Therapy Field School Guatemala. I am grateful to Pamela Pennington, Philip Wilson, Jonathan Maupin, Peter Rohloff, Gelya Frank, and Stephanie Roche for ongoing conversations and collaborations on what health in the Guatemalan highlands is and could be. Deep thanks to Nicole Berry, who went above and beyond to support the work of a junior colleague. Thank you to Lisa Munro, Amy Brown, Olivia Manders, Rebecca Watkins, and Juliana Kislin for editorial support and encouragement.

Thank you to my parents David and Becky Hall for sparking and supporting dreams, to Gari Clifford for sharing adventures and dreams of what could be, and to Bryce and Dorian for being dreams come true.

Most of all, I am indebted to so many Guatemalan friends and colleagues who have supported this work with their time, patience, love, insight, and expertise. Rosario, Mercedes, Nathaly, Juana, Pascuala, Eufemia, Mirian, *matyox chawe b'enaquel*.

All author proceeds from sales of this book go to Wuqu' Kawoq | Maya Health Alliance, a Guatemalan health organization dedicated to accessible health care in first languages for Maya communities.

Foreword

Waleska López Canu

My Story

I am a Kaqchikel Maya woman. I was born in Patzún, Chimaltenango, in the central highlands of Guatemala. I grew up in an Indigenous community in Mexico, exiled during Guatemala's armed internal conflict. After eighteen years, I returned to Guatemala.

My life in Mexico, despite shortcomings that could not begin to compare to those of Guatemala at the time, was full of learning. I was accompanied always by the inherited longing of my parents for an eventual return to Guatemala to contribute in some way to the development of our people.

I grew up hearing about the discrimination and oppression under which my people lived in Guatemala. I heard about the atrocities committed against us, the denial of accepting us, the Maya, as a living part of the people of Guatemala, and the lack of respect toward our way of life and thinking. I also grew up witnessing how the Mexican people held out their hand to my people when it was most needed.

I never felt like a foreigner in Mexico, but upon my return to Guatemala, I felt like a foreigner in my own country. The ignorance I had about my country and the loss of identity I had suffered by being displaced are things that I continue to recover and learn from. I am frustrated by the lack of love for their country and their own people that many Guatemalans have and by the despair that so many face.

My father is a farmer with a great love for the land, not only because it produces food but also because it gives birth to us as good men and women. My mother is a teacher, who has also been a seamstress, merchant, a caregiver, and a musician, with a great love for her family and her community. From them, I learned to love my neighbor.

My studies in medicine were not easy. I had to move a great distance from my village, and the only home that I had known, to a large city. Lack of money and access to technology, books, and easy transportation to hospitals made this transition difficult for me. More than that, I experienced the discrimination against women and against all of us who identified or had the appearance of being Indigenous. On one occasion, a professor told me to go home to make tortillas because I was never going to achieve a career. But here I am! The competition to finish with the best qualifications was a challenge. I had the good fortune of learning about community health and working in a rural area. This has always been my path.

When I came back to Guatemala, I had to join the national university, which I thought would be revolutionary, with opportunities for everyone so that all people could be educated. Instead, I collided head-on with a university that was full of the young bourgeoisie. They were the children of business owners and well-known professional elites and were totally unaware of the real health situation of their people. They had no interest in knowing it and much less in working to improve it. There were young doctors who did not want to go to certain placements work with "Indians." There were young doctors who made arguments like, "We should burn all these villages so that all the Indians who live there go to the city, and all the country's problems will be over." Even still, there are doctors and nurses who mistreat and belittle Maya-speaking patients. This makes me reflect on the long road still ahead to address the issues of health, racism, discrimination, and respect.

Health for the Maya

I worked nearly ten years in the extension of coverage program of the Guatemalan government's Ministry of Public Health and Social Assistance, first as a clinician and then as technical coordinator of six areas of the Chimaltenango Department. The program was good in theory, but in practice, it lacked everything except urgent needs. All of the problem solving, the immense physical effort of the work, and even the economic shortfalls of the health system became the responsibility of the workers themselves and the nongovernmental organizations that the government contracted to implement primary health care. Labor abuse, poor or no training, and a lack of capacity building were routine within the Ministry of Health. Programs were always created out of context and from an impractical view of what was possible, and the populations served were never considered in decision-making. We, the staff, were always blamed for poor outcomes. Even with these challenges, the program served hundreds of thousands of people and their health problems.

The Chimaltenango Department, despite being close to the capital city, has communities very far from any health service. Poverty and extreme poverty are very common in the communities we served in the government extension of coverage program. At that time, there were no roads or easily accessible transportation, and hospitals did not have the capacity to provide care for all the people who needed it. Traditional therapists, midwives, or culturally relevant programs were—and, I think, still are—viewed as mere embellishments. Of course, government health system employees have no say in decision-making or in the design of programs, but they are the ones who must comply with regulations, even when they are not applicable to our communities or our families.

The lack of respect for different ways of life and thought have added to the total lack of confidence in any public health service among the Maya people of Guatemala. The government system does not allow formation of an understanding relationship between doctor and patient.

Then, thirteen years ago, I found Wuqu' Kawoq The Maya Health Alliance. The mission, the vision, and philosophy of this nongovernmental organization dedicated to the provision of health services in communities in Maya languages was what I was looking for. I have worked with Wuqu' Kawoq ever since because I am able to direct health efforts, science, and resources to my people in a respectful, dignified, empathetic way that is shared by and with the Indigenous population. That is why I work here.

I started as a clinician in a nutrition program, serving children in communities in Chimaltenango and around Lake Atitlán. The complexities of managing malnutrition and the social determinants that we cannot solve are challenging, and yet we provide high-quality health services. Over time, I have helped build a diverse, versatile, well-trained team, primarily of Indigenous origin and, above all, committed to the health of the people we serve. We have learned a lot about ourselves as Maya, and we have gained a much broader vision of who we are, what we have lost, and what we must recover as we continue fighting for the dignity of life of Indigenous people.

The biggest challenge is that there are very few of us in Guatemala doing this work with this level of commitment to quality and this philosophy. We have shared the knowledge generated by our work with other organizations and with the government. However, the lack of political will and all the bureaucratic traps of social systems have meant that our programs, though successful, have not been adopted on a larger scale. This is both because of the costs they represent, but more importantly, because adopting them would require the deconstruction and reconstruction of ways of thinking and acceptance and trust between people.

At the local level, we have achieved so much. The government health centers, health posts, and regional offices know our work and understand that we have a real collaboration. Those who take care of patients and those who handle cases that are clinically and socially complex know and rely on our work. Unfortunately, they are not the ones who make the decisions at the highest level.

One of the efforts that I consider a success and a source of personal pride is the empowerment of my fellow women. Few women doctors want to work in rural areas and in research. My team includes nurses, nursing assistants, teachers, and social workers who have accepted the challenge of this work and who constantly continue to train—obtaining technical and clinical knowledge and building managerial and leadership skills. It is these women who are and will be the difference in the future.

About *Underbelly*

This book is a very honest, inquisitive, and, at times, uncomfortable look at the different realities found in Guatemala. In these pages, a very clear journey is made through the history of the country and the reason for the complexity of health issues in Guatemala. Talking (or writing) about diarrhea—from the perspectives of the political, economic, social, and cultural environment—is provocative, and it will resonate with similar cases outside Guatemala. This book expresses the way that inequalities are so marked by the lack of political will to make things different and how unfair it is that the lack of success of government programs or international cooperation falls on the shoulders of people in communities and frontline health service providers.

We cannot leave aside ancestral knowledge and the knowledge acquired through life experience. We must always build from a community's prior knowledge and understanding of health issues. This book addresses this issue in a very accurate and respectful way, emphasizing the importance of working together with the people of communities and not just for them, failing to include them in the processes of and decision-making about health projects.

It is first necessary to understand in order to reflect, redefine, recover, and build.

The Maya people cannot dismantle the relationship that exists between mind, body, spirit, and the environment. The situation of women, particularly Indigenous women, is complex. Therefore, health campaigns and the application of biomedical knowledge in communities must consider this context and work together. Maya women have always been responsible for the health care of their family. But they are positioned in society without authority, without resources, without time. Nevertheless, they always look for the best for their family.

Good intentions are not enough. Efforts must be coordinated and, above all, built jointly with the populations we serve. As Indigenous people, we do not like to live in the worst conditions and without rights. We have been pushed to do so. We do not want the crumbs of health services; we want high-quality care that is dignified and adapted to our culture and our day-to-day reality. Also, as Indigenous health providers, we want to be able to work toward these goals.

We cannot continue to expect people to be mere recipients of health services and programs that do not work for them and that they never wanted in the first place. We must be equal participants.

Underbelly is a journey from deep within the experiences of Guatemalan people. It presents a view from half a lifetime of discovery without judgment. It shares profound reflections and analyses of what health services and external global factors in Guatemala have been, what they have provoked, and what they could become. It emphasizes in a very respectful way how long-awaited health equity could be achieved.

Thank you for sharing this journey and this vision.

Waleska López Canu, MD

Medical Director, Wuqu' Kawoq | Maya Health Alliance
Tecpán Guatemala

Prologue

The sight of the black-and-white nun's habit encircling smooth, pale skin shocked me. I was already on edge from passing through three ancient doors that locked behind me, their heavy wood and iron fittings groaning back into defensive resting positions. I had last seen the warm, dark eyes of my friend Mercedes, now looking at me from the other side of iron bars, four years earlier in a village tucked up in the folds of the mountains of highland Guatemala. We were a long way from the small woodfire in her grandmother's kitchen where we last sat together.

Mercedes was seventeen when I moved to her village, and she rapidly became a trusted local guide and research assistant. She would patiently correct my garbled Kaqchikel, the Mayan language of the region, with smiles and giggles. She quietly told me the scoop on who was who and what was what in the village with a gentle voice that mirrored her attitude toward the world around her. The picture of youthful Maya beauty, Mercedes was petite with skin bronzed from hours of outdoor chores and farming and glossy black hair that was always neatly arranged with fashionable accessories. Her skinny frame was made curvy with a woven belt cinched tightly at the waist of her traditional *corte* (skirt) and a padded bra from the market under the intricately woven *huipil* (blouse) that she and her mother and sisters spent hours making. She thought my own clothes were unfortunate and manly, and she once insisted that I wear her clothes to a local wedding. After much laughter as her sisters and girl cousins were getting me arranged, Mercedes coquettishly pronounced, "There, now your husband will finally think you are beautiful! Take a picture!"

But for all her good looks, kindness, and energy, Mercedes did not quite fit in the village. As a lone *gringa* who had inexplicably left her husband

and home in *El Norte* to live in the village, I certainly did not fit either. I suspect this is what drew us together. As we spent hours tramping around the village on errands and conducting interviews and focus groups, she talked about wanting to leave. She was in an in-between phase that not many of her peers hold onto for long, having finished all the schooling available to her in the village but not yet married. The teachers at the local school spoke of Mercedes as a brilliant pupil, and she sometimes stopped by to help with the kids. But she talked about the future of women in the village with a sort of resigned inevitability—the babies that would come and keep coming, the washing, the work, the struggle to get enough. Once during lunch, her two young cousins fought over a piece of scrambled egg that had fallen to the kitchen's dirt floor, and I looked up to see Mercedes's eyes locked on mine. In that look, in that moment, I viscerally understood what she had been struggling to tell me. She wanted more—more food, more safety, more opportunities than the village could give her. No global health or development program, many of which had come and gone again, would fundamentally change the conditions of life there. She wanted out.

Mercedes attended the small Catholic church that sits on a hill in the middle of the village. Its brightly painted, concrete construction topped by a rebar cross and colored glass make the church stand out as a place apart in a village of more earthly colors and concerns. Mercedes went to the church for daily prayers, and I often tagged along to soak up the darkened quiet and moments to think, as the words of the Our Father and the Hail Mary in the language of the conquistadors echoed around us. Mercedes performed cleaning and organizational tasks around the church, her unattached availability making her vulnerable to favors asked by family, anthropologists, and the overworked traveling priest alike. The priest had spoken to Mercedes about joining a convent in Madrid, and her dreams had caught on this possibility. She talked of what it would be like to leave, to live in a church, to be in the world beyond the mountains. She talked of it so much and asked so many questions about travel that I left her my suitcase, bought on the cheap in Boston to carry my own dreams of becoming a medical anthropologist to Guatemala.

After I was no longer living in the village, Mercedes packed the suitcase and joined a cloistered order in Madrid. That gentle girl with steel resolve wore her beautiful huipil and plastic slippers for the last time on her first flight. I learned about the journey from her sister, but then I grew worried a few months later when her family had not heard from her. Her mother Maria and grandmother Flavia were becoming frantic, fearing their girl lost in a world they did not know. They did not have the full name of the convent but asked me to find Mercedes. I was living in England at the time, and I started calling a long list of convents in Madrid—looking for Mercedes, looking for mercy for her family in the big world beyond the village. I finally found the right convent and scheduled a visit by officiously claiming my status as family representative so that I could get an appointment with the Mother Superior.

When I arrived at the convent in central Madrid on the appointed day, the Mother Superior interviewed me at length about my intentions. I was finally allowed to pass through the gates and doors that have kept the outside world at bay for centuries, and Mercedes in her habit and robes was brought into a receiving room beautifully decorated but divided by bars. We both gasped in delighted recognition of seeing a familiar out-of-place and held hands through the bars. We chatted through pleasantries and updates sent from her family as the Mother Superior hovered and clucked her tongue when I ventured to speak a few words in Kaqchikel to the Mercedes from the mountains. "Listen to how good my Spanish is now," Mercedes said, and "you should see the food we have every day." Her figure had softened with such luxury, but she was confused when I mentioned the imposing palace nearby. "I think I saw it when I arrived from the airport, but it was dark," she said. The Mother Superior finally left us alone, and I immediately asked Mercedes if she was happy. I told her there are always choices and that I would bring her home if she wanted. But whose home? Whose choices? She smiled and said she was content.

This book is about choices and who gets to make them in global health. The limited choices available to Mercedes were shaped by systems of inequality that colonialism set in motion and contemporary neoliberalism maintains. Since the time of conquest, her Indigenous Maya community has faced centuries of violence and marginalization that have taken the food from their mouths along with their ways of life and access to land. Mercedes's choices were to promise her whole life to the practice of her faith under unknown conditions or to stay in poverty in the village. In fact, convents in Spain struggle to recruit novices, so they now look to young women from their former colonies in Latin America to fulfill duties to the faith forced on the Maya during conquest. It seems like an unfair choice, or not really a choice at all.

Mercedes's village in rural Guatemala was littered with the remnants of failed and forgotten efforts from a wide array of global health and development programs, their faded logos and hopeful slogans stuck to the sides of latrine stalls and chicken coops around the community. But the community never had the opportunity to choose what programs wound their way down the dirt road into their midst, and they certainly did not choose when distant program funding cycles and shifting trends meant those programs disappeared. Fundamentally, the lives of those left behind in the village and their health-seeking choices remain as cloistered as Mercedes's convent by the systems of inequality that have persisted across generations of marginalization and decades of health and development programming.

This book explores how the messy realities of global health efforts shape and constrain the choices of those whom they intend to help. The burden of childhood diarrheal disease is tragically mundane—a top-three killer of young children globally. Despite key successes, the glut of global health and development programming designed to address diarrhea over the past forty years has fallen short in many areas. Exploring local perspectives lays bare the choices, burdens, and barriers that global health programs create within recipient communities. Unmet needs, irrelevant offerings, and unintended consequences of globally conceived interventions are the underbelly of global health—hidden from view, unmeasured by indicators, obscured in reporting. Through this work, I hope to illuminate these hidden areas of global health, which I contend are the ones that matter most for people and communities as they navigate life and health-seeking in systems designed to their disadvantage.

The stories shared in this exploration of the lived realities of global health programs are those of real people—community members and leaders, health providers and administrators—but the stories are inevitably shaped by my own story and role. This book is based on more than fifteen years of ethnographic fieldwork, global health research, and program implementation in Guatemala. Early in my training as an anthropologist, I knew I wanted to understand how "global health" happened. I pursued professional training in global public health and initially felt like an outside observer struggling to understand how global health professionals think and work, but somewhere along the way I became one, too.

The asymmetrical power dynamics of global health, coupled with the fraught geopolitical and economic relationship of my home country of the United States with Guatemala, mean that my presence in Guatemala cannot be neutral. One of the joys of working in one region over such a long period has been watching friendships grow with people who started as research partners and realizing that our lives have become intertwined through birthday parties, celebrations, losses, and the lasting ties of godparenting that Guatemalans take very seriously. Yet, I have choices, privileges, and power that most of these colleagues and dear friends, including Mercedes, do not. Years of friendship and commitment to mutual work cannot erase these inequities. One of my challenges in sharing these untold stories from the underbelly of global health is recognizing and situating my own participation in the systems of inequality that made them happen. After all, I was the one, not her own family, who could go to find Mercedes in Spain, with my unearned access to the bits of paper and plastic that make travel possible. In considering my role within global health, I find guidance in the words of Guatemalan Nobel laureate Rigoberta Menchú: "What I give is only a tiny contribution, a grain of sand, but there is so much sand."[1] Revolutionary change comes through collective efforts, and we all have a contribution to make, however small. I firmly believe that we can use the immense resources of global health to center local communities as drivers of change toward health equity.

Introduction

The landscape of the central highlands of Guatemala is a Seussian vision of farmland with its patchwork quilt spread over the topography of a volcanic mountain chain. In the countryside, traditional crops of maize and beans seem to defy gravity as they cling to steep slopes where farmers struggle to eke out a subsistence. It is literally an uphill battle for most as population pressure and regressive land policies have pushed small-scale farmers further from solvency. In fact, 70 percent of the Indigenous Maya population experience chronic undernutrition.[1] To maintain a meager diet of corn tortillas and beans for their families, the rural poor journey into cities for wage labor in factories and agricultural processing plants, where they package nutrient-rich cash crops for export. They leave behind homes made of cinderblock or mud bricks or sometimes only reeds lashed together under sheets of tin roofing, in villages that frequently lack safe water and sanitation systems. The ancient, brightly painted American school buses that carry the rural poor into cities careen around hairpin turns and exhale clouds of exhaust on those left behind as they struggle up mountainsides with their human (and occasionally animal) cargo. They reach cities whose poor residents cannot boast a much better standard of living, with peri-urban shantytowns of rusted tin that could be anywhere in the world of the global majority yet somehow still manage to be uniquely Guatemalan—the marimba music and the scent of wood fires wafting overhead as residents go about the daily business of survival.

Guatemala has the unhappy distinction of being the second-poorest country in the Western Hemisphere, and it has one of the highest levels of income inequality in the world. Ten percent of Guatemala's population controls 90 percent of its wealth—the means, the mode, the whole *tamalé*.

Conflicts over economic policies favoring the wealthy and state marginalization of the Indigenous Maya population are not new to Guatemala; a thirty-six-year internal armed conflict left at least 200,000 dead and one million Guatemalans, or one-twelfth of the population, displaced. A United Nations commission found that the vast majority of killings were perpetrated by government forces against the Indigenous Maya and deemed these actions genocide.[2] Since the 1996 Peace Accords, Guatemala has settled into what can best be described as an uneasy peace. While the national army and guerrilla troops have ceased conflict, homicide rates increased from the early 2000s and have at times returned to the levels experienced during the height of the war. Income inequality, ethnic disparities, and government corruption—in short, the causes of the internal armed conflict—contribute to the current violence.[3]

Beginning in the mid-1990s when the armed conflict drew to a close, Guatemala became the recipient of a deluge of international development and global health funding. Eager to support the peace process and democracy, foreign governments provided funding for economic restructuring and infrastructural improvements. International nongovernmental organizations (NGOs) supported a cornucopia of health, education, and small-scale economic activities to help repair the shredded social fabric of communities. Airplanes filled with volunteer groups and church mission teams from the United States swelled the ranks of development efforts, and well-intentioned dollars flowed into the country. And the results were astonishing: not much changed. Despite all the money funneled into postwar Guatemala, sustained improvements toward income equality, health equity, and ethnic equality have been minimal.

Global Health in Neoliberal Times

Guatemala has a fragmented health system pieced together in the aftermath of genocide. It is underfinanced by a government that guarantees health as a human right to all but denies the humanity of many through inadequate provision of health and social services. This weak system is supplemented by a jumble of foreign-funded projects, from unregistered foreign volunteers who rove the countryside handing out basic supplies and medicines to multilateral government organizations that sponsor initiatives dependent on political will and economic climate. This book is about the experiences and choices of those left behind in local communities after the logoed four-wheel drives and air-conditioned vans return to urban offices and airports. I argue that in Guatemala—as in other places that struggle to shape a cohesive health system with heavy foreign aid, influence, and investment—countless uncoordinated global health programs shape and constrain local health-seeking choices in ways rarely captured by program evaluation metrics.

Global health itself is a slippery character. Much like the Guatemalan health system, "global health" is fragmented and multifaceted. Physician-anthropologist Paul Farmer, a thought leader of contemporary global health, famously remarked that "global health remains a collection of problems rather than a discipline."[4] Global health is a term used variously to refer to (1) the structures that *define* global health objectives, (2) the actors that *do* global health, and (3) the systems through which the actors and structures *deliver* global health. The structures of global health include in-country health systems; a vast array of local to large transnational NGOs, with the Gates Foundation poised as a dominant force in contemporary global health; bilateral government agencies such as the US Agency for International Development; and multilateral government organizations such as the World Health Organization and World Bank Group. The actors involved in global health are health providers, researchers, implementation teams, and policymakers at every level, of course, but they are also the populations framed as recipients of global health efforts. They are agentive and *do* global health more than any academic or bureaucrat. Finally, the systems of global health are perhaps the most difficult to pin down. We can look to supply chain logistics, implementation programs, and grant funding cycles as concrete examples of global health systems at work.

I am often guilty of using the term "global health" as a gloss for the less clear-cut systems behind global health actors and structures, those networks of power that are difficult to pin down but that we know are there because they leave fingerprints across the defining, doing, and delivering of global health. Often, the funding and, perhaps most importantly, the sources of that funding put the actors, structures, and systems of global health into motion and set the terms of engagement. However, having a shared understanding of the scope of global health work is essential.[5] An effort to define global health by Jeffrey Koplan and colleagues warns, "Without an established definition, a shorthand term such as global health might obscure important differences in philosophy, strategies, and priorities for action between physicians, researchers, funders, the media, and the general public."[6] This observation points to the critical challenge of having a shared mission across global health actors and structures to make our systems work to achieve desired (shared) outcomes. While defining global health remains elusive, the problems it seeks to solve—unrealized human potential and unnecessary human suffering—are ever present.

Further defining the dynamics of global health are the many terms available in bureaucratic politesse to indicate the haves and the have-nots: Global North/South; developed/developing; high-income/low and middle-income; global minority/majority.[7] For the discussion of global health systems and their broader geopolitical and economic contexts in this book, I use the terms high-income countries and majority world to intentionally foreground the prevailing wealth of a few countries within a supposed system of mutuality that perpetuates inequality.[8] In order to understand contemporary global health, we must first acknowledge that global health has its roots in the colonial enterprise. Its antecedents in colonial medicine and "tropical medicine" emerged through efforts to control, contain, and maximize the wealth to be extracted through the bodies of the colonized.[9] The origin story of global health further adds the moralizing paternalism of the "white man's burden" to the greed of the colonial system, a commingling of economics and self-interested morality that has persisted across the history of the field.

International health became codified in international policy and governance structures in the post–World War II era, as the United States and European victors rushed to (re)build a peaceful and profitable global economy. The human right to health was enshrined in the language of treaties and the missions of multilateral government organizations and transnational NGOs. Since that time, global efforts to improve the health of populations have cycled through various strategies and areas of emphasis, from technocratic approaches focused on specific infectious diseases to an emphasis on integrated primary care and back again.[10] Such efforts were renamed from international health to global health in the early 2000s in an attempt to reframe relationships rooted in colonialism and to center mutuality among high-income countries and the majority world.[11] Despite conceptual or at least semantic relationships of equity, the populations of majority world countries are still framed as the recipients of global health, and powerful, high-income countries work to reshape the health systems of the majority world in their own image. In the United States, our own shambolic, privatized health system fails to meet the human right to health of our population, but we have bought our way into the expert's seat in global health.

To understand contemporary global health, we must consider the meta-context of the contemporary neoliberal economy. Neoliberalism is built on the well-preserved ruins of colonialism—reminding me of the popular tourist markets in Antigua, Guatemala where Maya craftspeople sell their handiwork among the crumbled ruins of the Spanish colonial architecture their forebears were forced to build. Simply, the global flow of wealth—and the power that it wields—echoes patterns established in colonial times. The extraction of low-cost resources and labor creates profit for high-income countries and privation for majority world countries that leads to indebtedness and weak positioning in the global political economy. Unjustly enriched countries are then positioned to "save" the countries they have impoverished on their terms and when it suits them.

Neoliberalism is the particular form of capitalism that emerged in the late-twentieth century and has been marked by increased privatization and free-market principles.[12] The benefits of development are not equally distributed under any economic system, but neoliberalism has deeply enshrined disparities in the accumulation of capital and exclusion from it.[13] Private-sector and nongovernmental philanthropic funding have become key drivers of global health efforts as privatization has stifled government investment in social goods, including health services. Though certainly not identical to colonial times, contemporary global patterns of wealth and influence remain at an extractive homeostasis that we ignore at the peril of notions of equity.

The neoliberal turn of the global capitalist economy has indelibly shaped contemporary global health.[14] Global health programs can unintentionally perpetuate power imbalances between local populations who receive programs and the global health donors and actors who implement them.[15] Indeed, while the hopeful roadmap for "development as freedom" charted by Amartya Sen showed the way toward wider distribution of the benefits of development within neoliberal capitalism, freedom for those in the majority word too often means freedom to choose among inadequate options.[16] Neoliberalism is grounded in strategies of profit optimization and efficiencies that improve those profits. Incentives for production of a good life, including health, are shaped—limited—by these goals.[17] Within a pluralistic health care marketplace, care-seekers are required to be consumers, discerning for themselves which services to buy. Local communities often have little input in goal setting for the global health programs in which they are asked or even coerced to participate.[18] Health care becomes another commodity, and health system metrics become enmeshed with market metrics.[19]

In efforts to optimize (global) health, metrics have become our primary guides in shaping programmatic and funding priorities.[20] Numbers convert the messiness of life and global health into tidy metrics, but the lives of people and the realities of health-seeking get lost in the rounding.[21] With the expansion of global health as a neoliberal industry, the voices and perspectives of communities and recipients of global health are distal to decision-making.[22] Further, the competition spurred in the private sector to optimize profits in neoliberal economies spills over to the public and philanthropic sectors of global health as organizations compete for contracts, clients, and funds. As a result, cross-organization efforts to build cohesive, coordinated offerings within communities are disincentivized, as global health organizations of all stripes need to show measurable successes.[23] In responding to this myopic focus on metrics, I build on the work of other medical anthropologists who have argued for people-centered approaches to global health. Metrics are essential tools for illustrating trends and promoting transparency and accountability, but they must always be considered in conversation with the people and communities they purport to represent.[24]

The colonial history, neoliberal context, and metric-driven modus operandi of global health can feel abstracted from the *good* that global health seeks to do. Global health and development programs always have an underlying intervention philosophy—a moral rationale—for their implementation. Global health ethics advance utilitarian ideas about maximizing good and minimizing harm for populations as a collective.[25] Contemporary global health draws on an increasingly globalized social and economic value system centered on humanitarianism, which is itself inherently asymmetrical in terms of power, to enact human rights.[26] Just as colonialism relied on paternalistic moral justifications, the neoliberal economic system shapes our notions of morality, reifying notions of empowerment and agency while the accumulation of capital sets up some to be benefactors and others to be perpetual supplicants.[27] Yet the commitment to the human right to health pulls global health back to the universal good. To work toward the human right to health, social justice is the philosophical guide star of contemporary global health. For all of the forces of colonial legacies, structures, and power dynamics that would say otherwise, global health is guided by the principles of fairness, equity, and redistributive justice on which social justice is based.[28] Social justice animates action to repair our unjust systems of haves and have-nots and to push back against the neoliberal costs to our shared humanity.

The underbelly of global health stems from the neoliberal conceit that a pluralistic marketplace is an unequivocal win. Yet fragmented, pluralistic health systems make choices mandatory, replicating a neoliberal marketplace in which many are without the resources, financial and otherwise, to fully participate. Throughout this book, I look closely at the notion of choice, which is framed as freedom but is really an indicator of systemic failures to provide the right to health. I show how evaluation metrics and determinations of success in global health programs can elide the on-the-ground experiences of communities and even blame them for programmatic failures. I apply Pierre Bourdieu's concept of misrecognition, showing that inequalities are so pervasive that they are perceived as the natural order of global health systems.[29] Further, I introduce the idea of problematic gratitude, a relational by-product of neoliberal global health, in which the ever-shifting terrain of pluralistic health care landscapes requires money or connections (or both) to access health care. Fundamentally, I explore ways in which global health—its actors, structures, and systems—perpetuates the challenges it purports to fix. This is the underbelly.

Rosario's Impossible Choices

On a sunny afternoon in the small, remote Maya community of Panaj in the central highlands of Guatemala, I paid a visit to my neighbor Rosario.[30] Rosario's eight-month-old baby was very sick, with coughing and difficulty breathing in addition to ongoing episodes of diarrhea. While Rosario did her household tasks, the baby, a little boy named Efraín, spent much of his time swaddled on his mother's back or lying in a hammock made from tying the four corners of a grain sack to a roof timber with lengths of rope.

On this particular afternoon, Efraín was visibly dehydrated, with sunken eyes and labored, wheezy breathing. He whimpered but could not muster the energy to cry, and he did not turn his head when I firmly pinched his leg to check the severity of his dehydration. Rosario told me that Efraín had been sick for about a month, and I was shocked at his decline from a rounded bundle on his mother's back to this skeletal shadow of his former self.

Rosario was a strong and industrious Kaqchikel Maya woman in her mid-forties and worked tirelessly to support her nine children. She was brash and funny and down-to-earth. Her house was one of the humbler ones in Panaj, made of timbers and reeds lashed together and capped with scrap sheet metal. The house clung to the hillside, off a fork of the dirt road that runs through the village, and the dirt floor and open walls made it difficult to keep the house clean. It lacked piped water, so Rosario had to carry water in plastic jugs from a neighbor's hosepipe that received water pumped from an open-air lagoon. Rosario cultivated her family's small mountainside plot of land with her older children, growing as much of the maize and beans that form the basis of their diet as she could. Rosario's sole means of generating cash income was through selling her handwoven cloth in the municipal capital, and her husband occasionally sent money from his agricultural wage-labor on Guatemala's coastal plantations.

When a mobile health team had visited in the previous month, they told Rosario that Efraín had a respiratory infection and gave her a bottle of acetaminophen, apparently lacking an appropriate antibiotic for a patient so young. Rosario did not fully understand the directions they gave her on how to administer the medicine to Efraín, but she did her best. Rosario knew it would be another three weeks before the health team came to visit again. Two weeks after consulting with the doctor and nurse on the mobile health team, Rosario carried the baby forty-five minutes by foot to the neighboring village to visit the health post, staffed by a local community health worker. Despite holding a contract for a set number of hours per week with the government, the health post is known for erratic hours of operation and was closed when Rosario arrived.

Rosario considered making an onward trip into the municipal capital in the back of a pickup truck to visit the health center, the next rung on the primary health care ladder, but she did not have the money. She was also worried about her other eight children, whom she had left in the care of her fourteen-year-old daughter during the unsuccessful trip to the health post. She felt that the trip would probably not help Efraín, anyway. On the afternoon of my visit, I urged Rosario to take Efraín to a doctor and offered to pay for the trip or to make the trip with the baby myself.[31] Rosario responded, "No, I can't do anything else. Maybe it is better for my other children if this one dies. I can't take care of them." I left Rosario's house that afternoon with feelings of defeat: the baby was still sick, and his mother had little hope for the future of her family. Baby Efraín died two weeks later. Childhood illness, particularly diarrhea, is all too ordinary for the rural poor in Guatemala—a fact made real when Efraín was buried at the edge of the village graveyard in a section reserved for infants.

The Deceptive Simplicity of the Solution

I first came to Guatemala to study childhood diarrhea as a graduate student because I could not imagine why deaths like Efraín's keep happening. So many of the problems that plague our world are dizzyingly complex, but effective prevention of death from diarrhea just did not seem like it should be one of them. For children ranging from neonates through the age of five, diarrhea is the second-leading cause of death globally, a burden almost exclusively borne by populations in low- and middle-income countries.[32] The primary method of preventing death from childhood diarrhea is oral rehydration therapy (ORT), which has been a major global health intervention for more than fifty years. ORT involves giving an electrolyte solution by mouth to prevent dehydration. It is the simplest of global health strategies, requiring no complex supply chain or biomedical expertise to administer, and its flexible ingredients can be found in nearly every home. Only sugar, salt, and water—or even just the water that rice or plantains are boiled in—are needed to create an effective solution. The deceptive simplicity of oral rehydration and the underlying complexity of giving it to sick children is one of the most important global health stories. Before living and working in Guatemala, I assumed that effective ORT programs hinged solely on effective training of child caregivers—a simple issue of knowledge transfer. I was wrong. Training is only the preface to the true story of ORT, where seemingly simple instructions collide with social norms and role expectations, cultural patterns of childrearing and healing, and sociopolitical disparities in access to resources.

I was stunned a few years ago at a dinner party of academics in Oxford, England, when I heard someone across the room saying, "Imagine! Have you ever even heard of anyone dying from diarrhea?" in a critique of a new health system policy supporting rotavirus vaccine, which can help prevent infection from one type of severe diarrheal pathogen. Of course I had! The memory of Efraín was fresh and close to my heart, and I launched into a passionate explanation of just how much diarrhea affects the lives of millions of children around the globe, though they are distant from the privileged towers of Oxford and uncovered by benefits like the UK's National Health System. My husband seemed only slightly embarrassed as I pressed on with discussing diarrhea over dinner, knowing that I have been captivated and disturbed by the neglect of diarrhea as a dire cause of death of children since I began my training as a medical anthropologist and public health practitioner.[33] I have been told that this area of work is old-fashioned, meaning there are no new, exciting technologies to assess or discoveries to be made, and even that diarrhea is the "least glamorous" of global health concerns. In my view, the fact that diarrhea remains a persistent problem, despite decades of ORT education campaigns and work to improve water and sanitation systems, makes it deeply compelling, even more so because the solution feels as though it should be directly in our grasp.

The cases of diarrhea experienced by children in Latin America are innumerable and uncounted. Diarrhea accounts for approximately 8 percent of deaths of children under five in Latin America but over 18 percent of deaths in children under five in Guatemala.[34] Difficulties of application and uptake of ORT in areas with high infant and child diarrheal mortality rates are, by default, often attributed by global health programs to a disjuncture between the culture of biomedicine and the culture of the population targeted by ORT programs.[35] However, effective reduction of childhood deaths due to dehydration from diarrhea is not as simple as it seems. Within the Latin American setting, ORT campaigns have historically had limited success, although there were significant successes in response to improved water supplies prompted by the Millennium Development Goals.[36]

Guatemala has had active ORT programs for the past forty years and has seen reductions in diarrheal mortality. However, diarrheal morbidity and mortality continue to primarily affect Guatemala's Indigenous Maya population.[37] ORT campaigns in Guatemala and throughout Latin America have taken many forms, including distribution of packaged oral rehydration salts and teaching caregivers to make homemade solutions.[38] Although anthropologists have constructed taxonomies of Indigenous healing systems and their approaches to diarrhea, these are often framed in global health program design as barriers to implementation rather than understood as key existing resources. Further, longitudinal evaluations of the impacts of ORT campaigns on their targeted communities have been missing from the global health literature.[39] I set out to understand the gap between global health intentions and the on-the-ground realities of local communities in highland Guatemala.

The Guatemalan Context

Guatemala is a place of rich cultural diversity and extreme natural beauty, with lush volcanic landscapes and Mayan ruins wrapped in dense rainforests. Yet it grapples with entrenched ethnic conflict, extreme income inequality, and high rates of violence. While many of the challenges of engagement with global health and development programs in Guatemala are echoed across the majority world, they are also deeply patterned by Guatemala's unique context. Here, I briefly explore key elements of Guatemala's history that have shaped its own story with global health.

The Maya civilization's rise and decline then conquest by Spain mark a rich, complex, and painful start to what is now Guatemala. US neocolonial involvement in Guatemala has perhaps most influenced contemporary power dynamics and engagement with global health and development structures. Guatemala's internal armed conflict was set in motion in 1954, with the US-backed coup that overthrew leftist president Juan Jacobo Árbenz. Árbenz was elected in 1950, and in 1952, he implemented agrarian law reforms that began to redistribute unused lands held by the US-owned United Fruit Company. Land was given to 100,000 families to make subsistence-level farming possible and to remediate the land poverty that compelled the poor to work for large plantations for low wages. Lobbied by US economic interests in the country and worried about the approach of communism on its doorstep, the US government contacted exiled General Castillo Armas to stage a military coup. Using a shipment of Czech rifles approaching a Guatemalan port as pretext, the US government conducted air strikes in the two weeks preceding Armas's entry with US-organized troops from the Honduran border. Feeling hopelessly overpowered, Árbenz fled the country, and Armas quickly took power in June 1954.[40]

Armas himself was assassinated in 1957, by a presidential guard with leftist sympathies, pointing to the further fissures of Guatemalan politics and society. Conservative General Ydígoras Fuentes was then elected. Although he survived a military uprising in 1960, student and labor demonstrations in 1961 sparked the beginning of the guerrilla movements.[41] Fuentes was overthrown by the military in 1963, beginning a period of military dictatorships. In the 1960s, the United States sent Green Berets and directed a counterinsurgency campaign, and Guatemalan government death squads were formed. Throughout 1960s, the counterinsurgency was concentrated in Guatemala City, where university faculty and students, labor organizers, and activists were the primary targets until the conflict reached the countryside late in the decade. By 1979, the guerrilla groups, including the Organization of People in Arms (ORPA), Committee of Peasant Unity (CUC), and Guerrilla Army of the Poor (EGP), launched their first military offensives in the Ixcán area of northern Guatemala.[42]

In 1980, an Indigenous group from Quiché, a stronghold of the EGP, marched to the Spanish embassy in protest of army violence against civilians. Against the wishes of the Spanish ambassador, the Guatemalan army ignited and stormed the embassy, and all but one of thirty-five Indigenous protesters were killed. In 1981, the army counteroffensive began in earnest, which resulted in massacres and the destruction of more than 400 Maya villages by 1983. Following a sham election in 1982, counterinsurgency strategies escalated with the military coup of General Efraín Ríos Montt. Intense violence continued throughout the 1980s and early 1990s, with several government strikes to bring guerrilla movements under control, one further military coup, and two additional attempted coups.[43]

Forced disappearances, extrajudicial killings, rape, and massacres of Indigenous communities were key tactics of government and paramilitary forces. To control the Indigenous population and instill fear, government forces employed scorched-earth campaigns where villages and crops were burned to the ground, sometimes followed by forced resettlement in model villages where Indigenous communities could more readily be surveilled and controlled. Indigenous populations were forced to flee their homes and survive by hiding in the mountains. The government also enforced Indigenous community participation in civil patrols that sowed suspicion, forced complicity, and compelled informing on neighbors.[44] Key tactics of the guerrillas included kidnappings and ambushes, both often used to raise money and supplies. At least 200,000 people were disappeared and killed, and 1.2 million were displaced (10 percent of the population at the time) during the conflict.[45] At the conclusion of the conflict, the UN-backed Commission for Historical Clarification found that 93 percent of civilian killings were perpetrated by government forces and concluded that there was genocide—an attempt to physically destroy the Maya as an ethnic group—in Guatemala.[46] Peace Accords were formally signed in 1996, ending thirty-six years of internal armed conflict. However, the finding of genocide has been denied within dominant conservative political discourse since, and stealthier but pernicious ethnocide—the deliberate and systematic destruction of the culture of the Maya—has continued to attempt to erase the Maya from public life and force assimilation.

Since the Peace Accords, Guatemala has continued to face high rates of violent crime. Homicide rates were comparable to those at the height of the war in 2010, and while they have declined more recently, violent crime remains a serious concern and shapes everyday life.[47] Even development programs—the hopeful imagination of all that is possible in the Guatemalan context—are shaped by fear and security concerns.[48] Many national army soldiers became members of police departments following the Peace Accords, leading, in the views of many, to an increase of police brutality and corruption. As the postwar Guatemalan economy struggled to stabilize, there was an increase in narcotics trafficking through Guatemala to the United States. Though Guatemala itself does not produce large amounts of narcotics, drug cartels have used Guatemalan territory as an important clearinghouse for both product and money laundering, pocking the rainforests with clandestine airstrips.[49]

To say that the truth and reconciliation process remains incomplete in Guatemala is an understatement that echoes across the 500 years since conquest. A tiny yet powerful elite oligarchy still controls the systems of power and privilege that marginalize poor and Indigenous populations, though they are beginning to be supplanted by the newer money and power of narcotraffickers. Calls for transparency and accountability are unrealized.[50] Perhaps the most stunning evidence of the lengths to which Guatemala's elite would go to protect themselves was the murder of Juan José Gerardi Conedera in 1998. Gerardi, who founded the Human Rights Office of the Archbishop of Guatemala and oversaw the Recovery of Historical Memory project, documented atrocities committed during the conflict. Gerardi's report, along with that of another UN-backed truth commission, concluded that more than 85 percent of the violent crimes committed during the war had been perpetrated by the government and government-backed forces. Gerardi was found bludgeoned to death in his garage two days after release of the report.[51]

There has been limited prosecution of perpetrators of the genocide, though the past decade has seen movement of trials of crimes during the internal armed conflict in fits and starts. Ríos Montt, the military officer and dictator who became president of Guatemala and was widely held to be responsible for the worst human rights atrocities and massacres during the internal armed conflict, continued to be active in national politics through the mid-2000s. He was successfully prosecuted for genocide in 2013, only for the Constitutional Court to overturn the decision and continually delay the case on procedural matters until his death in 2018. In fact, the Guatemalan Congress voted to affirm there was no genocide in 2014, during the time of the Ríos Montt trial, and Attorney General Claudia Paz y Paz was removed from office early because of her role in leading the prosecution.

Corruption, stemming both from the traditional elite clinging to power and the influx of new money and influences from narcotrafficking and other illicit operations, is rife in Guatemala. Clandestine criminal networks and organized crime flourished as the Guatemalan armed forces were reduced and demobilized following the Peace Accords.[52] Criminals operate with relative impunity, and the justice system is ineffectual in successfully investigating and prosecuting crime. In 2006, the United Nations established the International Commission against Impunity in Guatemala (known as CICIG for the Spanish acronym). CICIG made important advances against corruption and filed more than 120 cases in the Guatemalan judicial system. CICIG proved so successful that its mandate was revoked in 2016 by Guatemalan President Jimmy Morales, who himself was under investigation for corruption. Guatemala ranks 149 of 180 countries in Transparency International's Global Corruption Barometer, and many of the judges and prosecutors involved in CICIG and other efforts to roust corruption have been forced to flee the country.[53] Despite a constitutional prohibition against immediate family members of those involved in a coup running for president, Ríos Montt's daughter Zury Ríos was at one point a frontrunner in polls for the 2023 presidential election. The inequalities that marked the civil conflict persist, if in new guises.

Social Suffering and Racism

Social suffering, as articulated and expanded by Arthur Kleinman, holds that human suffering can be caused by social forces, such as political, economic, and institutional turmoil, but also that such suffering transcends the individual.[54] The social suffering brought about by systemic racialization and marginalization enables intergenerational catastrophes of social exclusion, as we have seen across generations of Maya in Guatemala.[55] Poor Maya communities in Guatemala embody their low social status. They are short in stature due to chronic undernutrition. Their bodies are marked by diseases left untreated, and their families are scarred by the loss of loved ones to violence, illness, and hunger. Social suffering deeply affects not just the health of communities but also opportunities for health-seeking.[56] Because the Guatemalan government was responsible for the massacre of Maya communities during the internal armed conflict, the remaining Maya population often holds an understandable lack of trust in any government services, including health care.

Ethnic inequality and conflict underpin Guatemalan history and contemporary realities and will be explored throughout this book. Maya people like Rosario struggle to access the limited public services available primarily due to racism and its predictable sequelae of disenfranchisement and poverty. The ethnic binary of *ladino* or Indigenous typically used in Guatemala marks a fault line far more treacherous than those running beneath its many volcanoes. Ladino is used in place of the mestizo category common elsewhere in Latin America, but its emphasis on the mixture of Indigenous and European backgrounds is not taken on by most Guatemalan ladinos, who frequently emphasize and creatively trace their European heritage.[57] Ethnicity and power, both economic and political, have a direct relationship in Guatemala: it is a "pigmentocracy" in which the lighter your skin, the closer you are to the apex of society.[58] The horrific violence of "whitening" the population through the rape of Indigenous women by ladino men was historically viewed by the ruling white elites as virtually a public service.[59] Racism in Guatemala does not hide, but it has hidden impacts on personal identity and public life for the Maya placed, with few exceptions, at the bottom of society's pyramid.

The extremely wealthy, white oligarchy who have essentially controlled Guatemala since the time of conquest fiercely maintain the social order, in part, through the racial minoritization of a majority of the population.[60] One member of this elite group told me in conversation:

> Our Indians are lazy. They don't want to work, and they don't really want things to change. Other countries [in Latin America] have it better because they got rid of all of the Indians early on. We Guatemalans have kept trying to integrate them into society, but we've been trying for hundreds of years.

This interlocutor has dedicated much of his life to public service, sits on the board of multiple philanthropic foundations, and seemingly saw no contradictions between these undertakings and his stark othering of the Maya. In this conversation, I felt the use of the offensive term "Indians" was meant to elicit a reaction from me, a foreign researcher out of place at a fancy party in Guatemala City, but I have no doubt that he uses it regularly. I grew up in the US South and am no stranger to the displays of racism that my own whiteness makes me privy to through the unwelcome assumption of shared views. This man thought I would understand his monolithic contempt for the Maya because we were both racialized as white. He went on to argue that the Maya want immediate benefits from the government and development groups but do not want to be bothered beyond that. "They don't really want things to change," he said. The violence of such overt and pervasive racism throughout Guatemalan society transmutes social participation into multivalent social suffering for Maya populations in Guatemala.

The Research

In conducting the research for this book, I was my own flawed, embodied self. I am a middle-class, cisgender, heterosexual white woman from Tennessee in the southern United States. I am a medical anthropologist. I am a global health practitioner. I inevitably bring all of these identities and more to my work in Guatemala and beyond. Where global health is a field of urgency, anthropology is a discipline of patience. My work sits at the intersection of the two. I apply the research techniques of anthropology to the design and evaluation of global health programs. Anthropology is rooted in building deep understanding of places and phenomena, most often through participant observation or simply living among and being a part of the communities of study. This takes time to achieve. Global health strives to be responsive to ever-evolving real-world conditions through evidence-based practice, but overreliance on quantitative data can obscure the real experiences of real people. This is where the contextualized knowledge of anthropologists can play a role.

My career as an academic medical anthropologist coupled with work as a global health practitioner—actively working with communities to develop and implement health programs—has given me a wide-ranging view across the research and implementation spectrum in global health. Academic work often focuses on after-the-fact analysis and critique more than it offers generative ideas for new approaches. Critique is essential but can lose sight of the imperative to *do* something, since the human right to health compels us to act, even if imperfectly. On the other hand, global health actors can become so caught up in the doing and the need to make an impact that they fail to consider that their real impacts may be harmful.[61] The urgency often felt in global health work can lead to cavalier attitudes and brushing aside ethical concerns with a myopic focus on a predetermined goal.[62]

In working across the academic and practitioner divide, I have had the opportunity to work in many different settings where global health takes place, from rural villages to national ministry of health offices to World Health Assembly meetings. My expertise alone did not earn my access to these rarefied settings; unearned prestige had a lot to do with it. I have trained and worked in high prestige institutions in high-income countries, and I am very aware of the doors this has opened for me but that remain closed for others. Throughout this work, I attempt to position myself— including my biases and failings—in relation to what I have learned about global health and its differential reach across populations. I draw on my many years of research and implementation experience to consider how global health really happens and to highlight how community voices can be made more central.

This book is an ethnography of global health, drawing on long-term ethnographic research to intentionally draw linkages across local to international levels. Ethnography is centered on participant observation, the hallmark method of anthropology in which the researcher lives, works, and joins in the activities of the study community.[63] This method enables a rich understanding of life and perspectives from within communities, but it is also fraught with challenges of authenticity and the ethics of engagement in everyday life as an outsider.[64] I worked to carefully explain my goals in all research communities and to not just ask my own preformed research questions but to ask my interlocutors what questions we should be asking together.[65] This approach has shaped the data that I present in this book as well as the co-design model that I now apply to global health program development.[66] I first lived in Guatemala for a continuous period from 2006 to 2007, conducting the ethnographic research on childhood diarrheal disease that forms the foundation of this book. I conducted participant observation in a variety of communities, homes, and health care settings. Additional research methods in my ethnographic toolkit included in-depth interviews with community leaders, health system stakeholders, and parents; focus-group discussions with mothers; household and caregiver surveys; and countless informal conversations.

Since that initial long-term fieldwork, I have typically spent an average of two months of each year living and working on global health projects in Guatemala. I conducted a two-year study of the implementation of zinc supplementation with standard treatment for childhood diarrheal disease.[67] For eight years, I have been a team member on a project to improve the perinatal continuum of care for rural Maya women who face some of the highest maternal mortality rates in the Western hemisphere. This began as a clinical trial that tested a low-cost perinatal monitoring toolkit co-designed with Maya midwives, and it has continued as the standard of care for the partner health organization in the region.[68] I have additionally worked on research and implementation projects on water quality, nutrition, short-term medical missions, education, migration, and health systems strengthening. I am in-country director of a global health field school in Guatemala, which has given me the opportunity to build institutional relationships with Guatemalan universities, advocacy networks, and community organizations. Projects undertaken by the field school, primarily program evaluation work, are identified as needs by partner organizations and conducted collaboratively between students and local partners. All of this research and implementation experience informs my perspectives and the data shared in this book. Mostly, it is my time spent living, being, and learning within Guatemalan households and communities that has shaped my understanding of how global health happens in people's lives.

In this book, some names of people and places are anonymized to protect participants. These decisions were made with individual participants and communities across time and through multiple discussions of whether they wanted their thoughts and experiences directly attributed.[69] I have discussed portions of this ethnography with those directly depicted, members of communities included, and other global health and development practitioner-scholars over years to shape the analysis of and lessons learned from the rich ethnographic data that we constructed together.[70] This ethnography is a collaborative work. I also use more photos of people and interior community spaces than is common in ethnographies. The photos selected support my goal of accurately depicting life in highland Guatemala, but I also believe they represent the agency of my interlocutors. I am the photographer, but the photos were selected with participants according to how they wish to depict themselves and their spaces, occupations, and care-seeking.[71]

The Research Setting

Living in a Rural Maya Community

Rustling sounds under my head that I desperately wanted to ignore meant the start of the day. It would only be a chicken, rodent, or the occasional dog snuffling around on the earthen floor underneath the wooden bed frames stretched with rope. These were the sleeping arrangements to which we retired the night before, lying under piles of blankets in the early evening as temperatures fell with the sun. The metal grain silo in the corner of the room drew the animals, hopeful for a few dropped kernels, just as the promise of the warmth of the fire drew me into the new day. I exchanged sweatpants for trousers, slid out of bed, slipped on my shoes, and creaked open the door—the *tsk-tsk-tsk* of the broom against the hard-packed dirt of the patio a gentle rebuke that the day had started without me. The room I shared with Mercedes, her younger sister Silvia, older sister Juana, and their mother Maria was already empty even though dawn was just beginning to break, the faint light stealing through the crevices where tin roof meets earthen bricks.

Crossing the patio and stepping into the corrugated metal kitchen shelter, I heard the *slap-pat-pat-pat* of tortillas being made and the bubbling of water for tea or Nescafe, if someone had been feeling flush at the market. The piney smoke from the open fire smarted in my eyes, filling my nostrils with present-tense nostalgia. Doña Flavia's kitchen fire was the center of the world, an *axis mundi* around which we all revolved. It was a world circumscribed by the steep mountains that keep the village a world unto its own. The twisting, rutted dirt road and the mobile phone in Doña Flavia's apron pocket were the threads that kept us tethered to the outside world.

Other threads of love and longing were less susceptible to the whims of the rainy season: Estrella's thoughts of a husband away in El Norte working for more than three years; Mercedes's dreams of moving to Spain as a nun—a fanciful idea planted by the traveling priest; and Juana's plans for something more—school, work, whatever the city could bring. The village is a forty-five-minute walk past its nearest neighbor whose name Simejuleu means "edge of the world" in Kaqchikel and always seems like a dare. Daily life over-the-edge began and ended around the kitchen fire.

Doña Flavia's household included three female-headed family units that each had a sleeping room and shared the kitchen, water basin, and latrine. Flavia herself was on her own—her husband and a son were killed in the internal armed conflict, and her other children were grown. Her daughter Maria's husband was also killed, and she was raising her three teen daughters Mercedes, Juana, and Silvia to be strong and independent. Estrella, Flavia's daughter-in-law, had her three young kids to manage while her husband earned their future in the United States. Though each of the women had her own challenges, they were all proud to be succeeding as a household of women—no small feat in patriarchal Guatemala. Flavia's age, life experience, and level head meant that men and women in the village frequently asked her for advice, and she routinely hosted Indigenous village council meetings by the warmth of the fire with the fortification of a maize *atol* porridge. The fire was where plans were made, dreams were hatched, and problems were solved. The women were known as organizers—of the women's weaving cooperative, of efforts to get a middle school in the village, and very quietly, of more political efforts.

This household of women sits at the center of the village and near where the biweekly microbus stops to pick up passengers ready for the hopes and challenges of the municipal market. I realized after some weeks of living in the village that my status as a *profesora* gave me unearned access to a ride in the back of the pickup truck that brings teachers from the municipal seat out to the village primary school each morning and takes them home at midday. The first time I visited the village with a friend from the weaving cooperative, the teachers, hired for their ability to speak Kaqchikel as a first language and to understand local culture, warned me off by describing the hardships and isolation of the community. As the pickup careened around hairpin turns and through clouds of dew-filled morning air, I took in the lush trees and humble homes against a backdrop of breathtakingly vertical cultivated fields. I did not yet know how Doña Flavia's plastic slipper-clad feet would fly up the path to her own plot, leaving me breathless as I struggled to keep up. On this first trip, schoolkids spotted me in the back of the truck and ran in the river of dust left in our wake like minnows in a slipstream. I could only smile and laugh with them as they called out *kaxlan* in Kaqchikel, which translates generously as "foreigner" and more uncomfortably as "conquistador." I was far from the parts of Guatemala where hordes of tourists and well-meaning do-gooders from abroad make for unremarkable sights. I brought my own foreign gaze to the localized reality of 500 years of violent marginalization and the challenges of health-seeking for rural Maya communities, but it is Rosario, Mercedes, Flavia, and all the people I came to know within the communities who have seen and lived it all.

Village Life in Context

Panaj is a small village of 2,000 Kaqchikel Maya inhabitants, or about 150 families, in the Comalapa municipality of the Chimaltenango Department, nestled in the mountains of Guatemala's central highlands. Chimaltenango has been called the beginning of the real Guatemala, meaning that it is the gateway to the west of Guatemala City where departmental populations become majority Maya (see figure 0.1).[72] The department's total population is about 600,000, of which approximately 70 percent are Maya, primarily Kaqchikel.[73] The department is divided into sixteen municipalities, and the city of Chimaltenango is the departmental capital, forming a regional hub for government, health systems administration, and NGOs. The violence of the armed internal conflict during 1970s and 1980s was fierce in the department, health and development efforts were seriously forestalled, and economic development was slow to come to this part of the highlands.[74] Memories of the violence are ever-present and continue to shape the lifestyles and attitudes of the population of Panaj and throughout the Chimaltenango Department.

Panaj is about an hour by truck on the lone dirt road to Comalapa, the municipal seat. The households that form the village lie on the two steep sides of a small valley (figure 0.2). At the center of Panaj, where the road forks uphill to dispersed households and downhill to the primary school, are two tiny shop windows that open onto the street from private homes. Further down the road is the brightly painted Catholic church, and the primary school marks the end of the village. Most residents of Panaj socialize

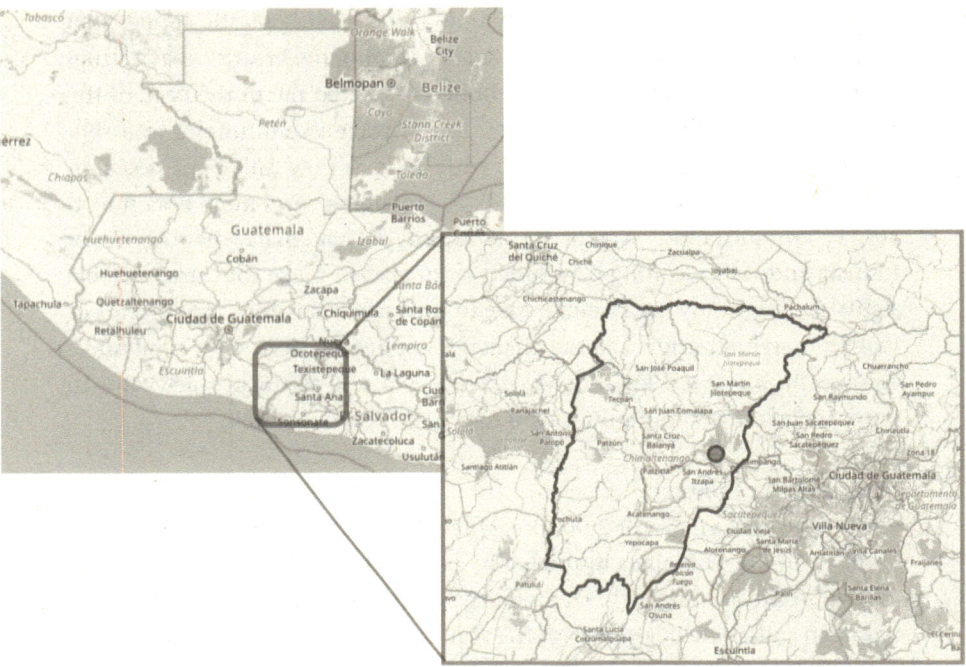

Figure 0.1

Map of Guatemala, Chimaltenango Department inset. Adapted from OpenStreetMap: https://www.openstreetmap.org/relation/214715#map=10/14.6341/-90.8219.

primarily within their extended family group. Trips to the Comalapa market and, less often, the city of Chimaltenango are significant events. Most homes in Panaj are made of homemade mud bricks and caned walls with tin roofs (figure 0.3). A few families now have homes made of cinder blocks and with concrete floors, construction made possible by remittances sent home from family members working in El Norte in the United States. Most families have a small separate lean-to structure for cooking over a wood fire, although the poorest members of the community build their fires in their primary living space. No family has a constant source of piped water, but the intermittent water supply pumped from a nearby lagoon is shared in turns organized by the village council. About half of the families in the village have basins for holding water, while the others use water out of plastic barrels and tubs.

Every family in Panaj has a plot of land that they farm for subsistence, primarily relying on corn augmented by beans, though registered land

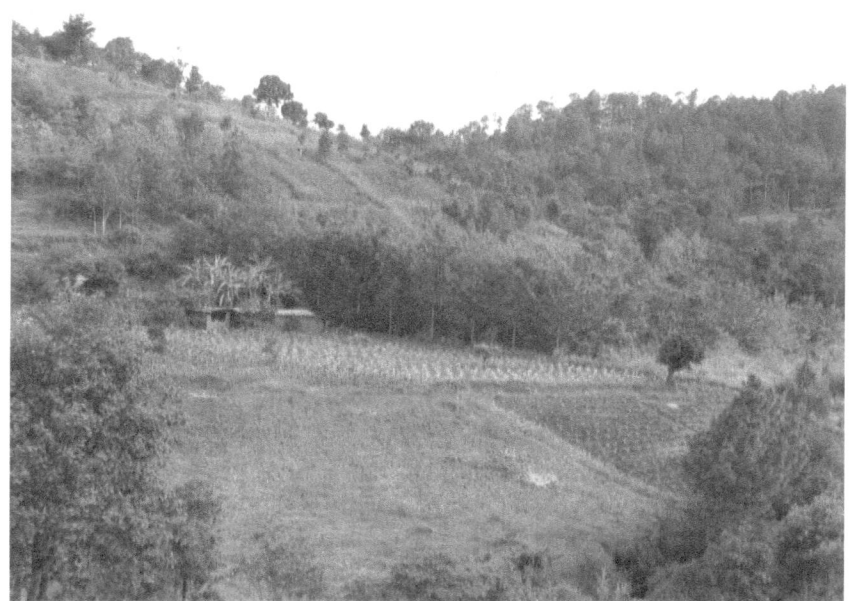

Figure 0.2
The landscape of Panaj.

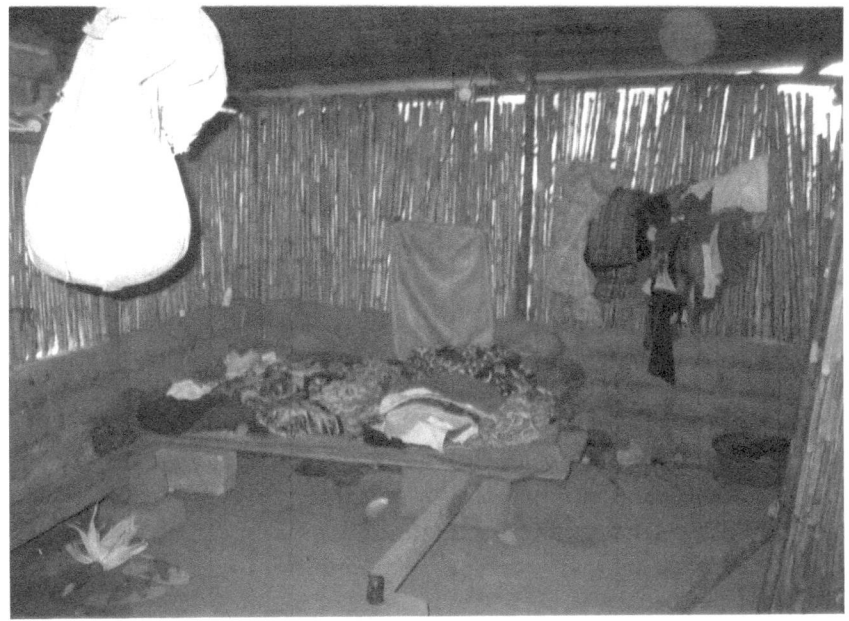

Figure 0.3
A typical household in Panaj.

ownership is uncommon. Some families have larger and more desirable plots of land, and they are able to grow cash crops for export. Raspberries were a common cash crop during my fieldwork, though they were a new and risky enterprise. However, many families' plots of land are too small to sustain the family, and men often have to seek wage labor in Guatemala City, the coastal plantations, or though migration to the United States. Women commonly live in extended family households, like Doña Flavia's, with the men absent for long periods of time. The women cultivate subsistence crops, and some take part in a weaving cooperative through which they sell their handicrafts for export to the United States. As we saw in Rosario's story, there is no health facility in Panaj. A government health service visits monthly, and the closest health post, staffed only by a community health worker, is a forty-five-minute walk away. The nearest staffed health facility is in the municipal capital of Comalapa.

Towns as Vital Hubs of Life and Resources

Research presented in this book also centers on two towns in Chimaltenango Department: Comalapa, the closest town to Panaj, and Acatenango, a primarily ladino town surrounded by communities of Maya coffee farmers. Comalapa is a large town of 25,000 people, but many local residents call it a village in reference to its Indigenous identity. Comalapa was a hub of organizing and activity during the armed internal conflict and continues to be a hub of Kaqchikel Maya culture, activism, and identity. At its entrance, Comalapa, known throughout Guatemala for its artists and distinct style of painting, has beautifully painted murals depicting the story of the town that pass across the entrance to the ornate cemetery and carry on into the center of town. The murals include graphic depictions of Maya villagers being tortured and murdered both by guerrillas and army soldiers during the conflict, perhaps an attempt to remind residents that history is complicated. With a fountain depicting the face of Marxist revolutionary Che Guevara, who passed through Guatemala in 1953, Comalapa is still more openly political and pro-Indigenous rights than most Guatemalan towns. Several NGOs, including microcredit institutions, agricultural development programs, educational enrichment programs, and health initiatives, are active in Comalapa.

Comalapa's central square bustles with activity and serves as a focal point for public life (figure 0.4). Municipal wash basins are available for those who

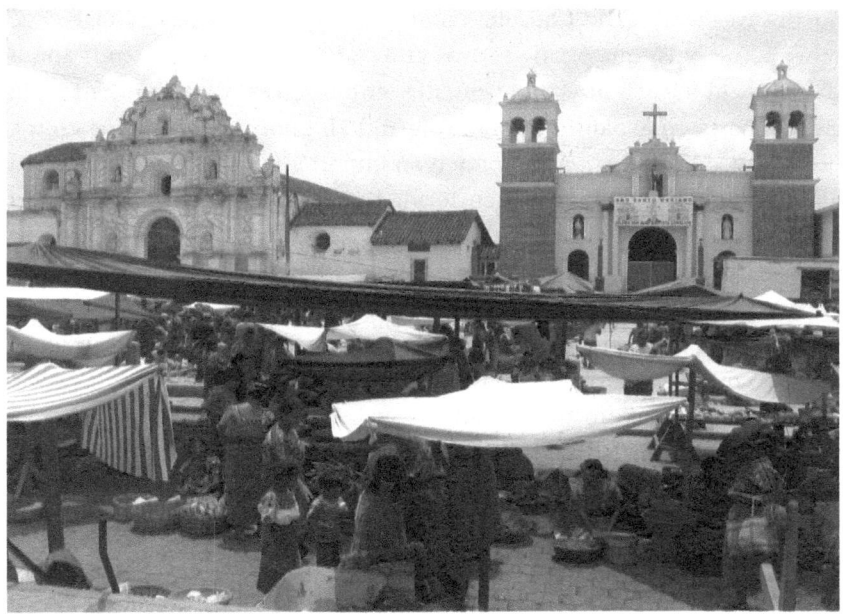

Figure 0.4
Comalapa's central market.

do not have running water in their homes. Most afternoons, these basins are crowded with Kaqchikel Maya women washing clothes, their hair, and the occasional child and catching up on the latest news. The twice-weekly market is central to Comalapa's economy, where individual vendors and local businesses trade with the many villagers who come from surrounding communities like Panaj. Most of Comalapa's surrounding communities practice small-scale subsistence agriculture. Further, many Comalapa men and some women commute daily into Chimaltenango or Guatemala City to work as wage laborers in offices, factories, construction, and domestic service.

Also a municipal seat like Comalapa, Acatenango is a small town of 10,000 people situated on the side of a (sporadically active) volcano of the same name. The road climbing the mountains to reach Acatenango offers breathtaking views of the patchwork of sharply inclined *milpas* or farm plots. Acatenango itself is primarily a ladino town, although the surrounding villages are Kaqchikel Maya. The town has a small central square where the weekly market is held on Sundays and youth basketball games are held on the weekends. The Catholic church and municipal offices face each other across this square. The formal grid of the town only extends about three blocks in each direction from the central square, though recent rapid growth has seen expansion of housing and an informal settlement on the northwest side of town. Autonomy is an important element of Acatenango identity, shaped by its experience during the internal armed conflict. Local people recount with pride how the guerrillas and the army were both kept out of Acatenango because the townspeople formed a strong guard against outside infiltrators.

Acatenango's economy and identity center on the production of high-quality coffee for export, processed through a local coffee cooperative. Many wealthier ladino town residents own small plots of land that they use for growing coffee. However, most coffee production occurs on large plantations, owned by absentee ladino owners and managed by ladino supervisors. The Kaqchikel Maya workers and their families often live in plantation-owned housing, which consists of one dirt-floored room and

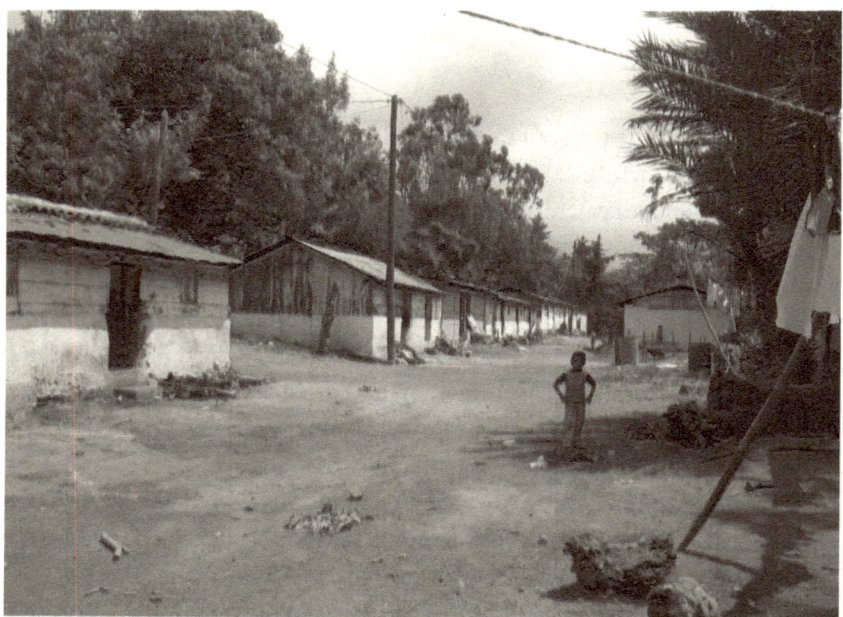

Figure 0.5
Coffee plantation housing in Acatenango.

bedstead per family (figure 0.5). Living conditions on the plantations are typically poor, and the cost of housing is often so high that workers become indebted to plantation owners over the course of the year before the harvest comes in, which compels them to continue working (and living) at the plantation. Acatenango and Comalapa, as municipal seats, both have staffed health centers, though the hours of operation and primary care services offered are variable. Some basic health services are occasionally available on the Acatenango plantations, but they are fee-for- service.

City Infrastructure, Resources, and Realities

The City of Chimaltenango has a population of 67,0000 and is the government seat for the Chimaltenango Department. The city was leveled in 1976, when it was at the epicenter of a devastating earthquake that demolished its traditional architecture of whitewashed adobe and red-tiled roofs. After the earthquake, an influx of international aid and development agencies helped rebuild Chimaltenango, transforming it into a city of cinder block and sheet metal.[75] The central square has the colonial style common to most Guatemalan towns, with the cathedral, municipal buildings, and police station arranged around a central park (figure 0.6).

Chimaltenango sits on the Pan American Highway and is a major transportation hub for Central America as well as Guatemala, with trucks clogging its highway bypass and providing business for its many sex workers. The primary form of public transportation in Chimaltenango and between all major towns and cities in Guatemala is the fleets of privately owned, brightly painted old American school buses. Passing through town on the highway, bus driver assistants lean precariously out of the buses, shouting the destination so that waiting passengers can find their way. These buses are often impossibly full, with standing room only and goods and animals tied to their roofs on market days.

The economy of Chimaltenango depends on commerce and the related service industries that result from being the commercial hub of the region. Chimaltenango is also fringed with factories, which churn out everything from textiles to building supplies. Central American and American chain stores and restaurants have made it to Chimaltenango, creating appealing opportunities for recreation for families in surrounding areas. Chimaltenango also has two large local markets: one whose stalls primarily sell fresh produce and meat and another, near the central bus terminal,

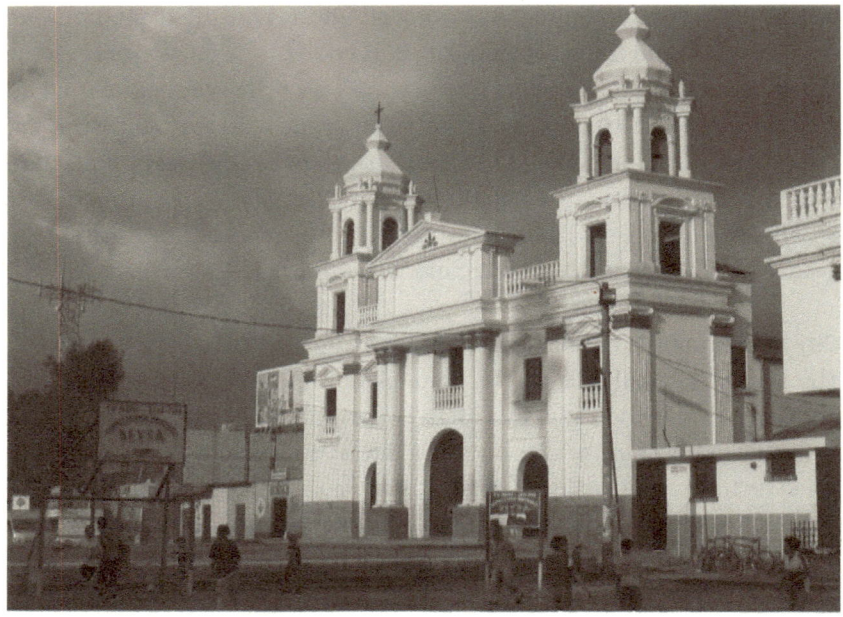

Figure 0.6
The cathedral and central square of Chimaltenango.

that specializes in nonfood merchandise, such as plastic goods, shoes, and electronics.

Crime rates are high in Chimaltenango, and since the 1990s, gang and narcotrafficking activity has become common. Gangs have also become a default explanation for violent crime and a way of maintaining community cohesion. For example, when a young man was robbed and brutally beaten on the corner of the block where I lived in Chimaltenango, the entire neighborhood seemed to find comfort in the explanation that it was "only" gang activity and that no one from the neighborhood was implicated. The violent history of the internal armed conflict and the high rates of current violence shape most aspects of city life in Chimaltenango.

As the department's capital and largest city, Chimaltenango has a government health center for primary care as well as a hospital that receives referrals from the department's outlying health posts and centers. Designed in the aftermath of the internal armed conflict, the terms of the Peace Accords put pressure on the government to reach rural communities with health services and to provide health and social services in Maya languages.[76] It has a tiered structure with primary care on the bottom and tertiary care on top. Guatemala's health system is a thing of beauty—on paper. However, in practice, provision of primary care to rural communities has been uneven and rarely delivered in Maya languages. Tertiary care is confined to urban centers, and specialty and referral hospitals are clustered in Guatemala City.[77] Deep disparities exist between urban and rural, ladino and Maya, and wealthier and poor segments of the population in terms of who can receive timely, quality care in the government health system. As a result, a wide array of philanthropic and private-sector offerings have emerged to fill the gaps of the government health system.

Book Overview

Chapter 1 further explores how trends in global health and the local realities of Guatemala have led to the application of a stopgap measure like ORT as a long-term, inadequate solution. Since 1979, the World Health Organization has promoted ORT as an effective treatment against the often-fatal dehydration and malnutrition in children with diarrhea, and we have seen incredible successes from this strategy. As we have learned, ORT is a simple solution, but it is not easy to use consistently and effectively. In chapter 1, I explore how low rates of ORT use are often attributed by default to the culture of those targeted by ORT programs, displacing blame for program failures onto recipient communities. Childhood diarrhea becomes framed as a choice made by the poor rather than a systemic failure. Yet, diarrhea continues to be a critical health concern because its underlying causes, primarily lack of clean water and sanitation systems, have not yet been adequately addressed by public systems. Within the Guatemalan context, the cascade of consequences from lack of water and sanitation infrastructure to limited health services and impracticable, even moralizing, ORT campaigns to poor child health outcomes serve to further entrench racial inequality and stigma.

As caregivers of children, women are the target audience of global health programs, but they often have limited power to implement suggested practices, particularly because of Guatemalan cultural norms of male control of finances and patriarchal limits placed on female travel. Chapter 2 explores the ways in which global health programs can increase the burdens of gender inequality. In Guatemala, women, particularly Indigenous Maya women, are targets of violence at the national political level, within local communities, and at home. These injustices are misrecognized as the natural order of things. Women's position in society (dis)enfranchises them, shaping their access to the resources, information, and mobility required to effectively navigate the health care system. The unequal position of women in society directly affects their agency in childrearing and health-seeking for children, and it shapes how they must choose to prioritize scant resources and navigate exclusionary systems. Finally, this chapter revisits the concept of "hygiene" with an intersectional lens to unpack the castigation of mothers as "unhygienic" when their children have diarrhea.

Even if you have the autonomy to seek health care in rural Guatemala, access is not guaranteed. The knowledge of how to gain access to the formal health system can be confounded and confused by an ever-changing array of available services and programs for many in Indigenous populations in Guatemala. In chapter 3, I explore the pluralistic care-seeking landscape for the rural Indigenous poor. We will see that marginalized populations with few economic resources are embedded in a health system in which they recognize that better treatments and services are available but not within their reach. I argue that choice is conflated with freedom—but the choices that are available and accessible are shaped by historical legacy and contemporary inequality.

In particular, I examine the impacts of violence, both remembered and continuing, on utilization of the health care system. Operating from a position of suspicion and fear, rural residents often hide from health teams making their monthly village rounds and, occasionally, even respond with violence. Though they lament the fact that their urban counterparts have superior health service options, some rural residents also say that health workers should not "force" them to take any vaccine or treatment they do not want because they want control of their own bodies. Health workers tell their own "war stories" of being chased by villagers with machetes and how they approach rural households with rocks in their fists to safeguard against the guard dogs that are sometimes turned against them. The low usage rates of the health system are then pointed to as a rational basis for limiting the expansion of government health services. By examining rural Indigenous attitudes toward the Guatemalan health system, this chapter considers how physical violence begets and sustains the structural violence that limits the autonomy of communities and choices of individuals within them.

In chapter 4, I delve into the interstitial spaces that shifting health and development programs create for the growth of private-sector health services and commodities, which further introduce the opportunities and burdens of choice. Quasi-pharmaceutical pyramid schemes doubly burden poor populations by recruiting them as low-level vendors with promises of huge profits and by misinforming them as product consumers. Social obligations and aspirations encourage the purchase of expensive "miracle" products, whose indications always happen to match customers' symptoms. In this chapter, I investigate the consequences of untrained vendors dispensing health advice along with dubious products in the cases of childhood diarrhea. I also explore individuals' choices and power over their own bodies and their health care by prioritizing costly, private-sector services. We will visit poor households that frequently display aged bottles of an expensive ORT product as a significant social symbol of the ability to provide for their children, even though those children have never received an adequate dose of the solution. We will see how prestige products and services reinforce the notion that health equals wealth but too often yield empty promises of the high quality of care for which they are an illusory proxy. This creates a highly neoliberal experience of social suffering, in which segments of society are both disadvantaged and taken advantage of in an unfair health care marketplace.

Chapter 5 moves from a focus on individual choices and actions within the fragmented, pluralistic Guatemalan health care system to think more deeply about the global health and development structures that have helped create this system. In Guatemala, as elsewhere in the majority world, an aura of frustration and futility overhangs many development workers, local and foreign, NGO and government alike. I assert that the multiplicity and lack of coordination of health and development programming leads to an active inertia, where despite a great deal of activity, little substantial, sustainable change is achieved. Expenditures of material and human resources that fail to create change are not just programmatic failures but also cause harm by abetting entrenched inequalities. Guatemalans targeted by various global health and development efforts have become jaded—taking what they can from new programs with the knowledge that they will soon be gone and replaced by others. These systemic failures are not unique to Guatemala; rather, they are repeated around the world in neoliberal global health structures and systems. By failing to reckon with unequal global (neo)colonial socioeconomic power dynamics, global health risks being a change in name only from colonial medicine and the patterns of global inequality it set in motion.

Above all, despite the challenges that I describe, I am optimistic. In the conclusion, I highlight pivotal points at which we might apply pressure within global health and development structures to move toward lasting change and effective collaboration with local communities. In particular, I introduce the co-design approach, which centers community priorities and practices in the development of global health programs.

1 Oral Rehydration Therapy and the Not-So-Simple Solution to Diarrhea

When children have diarrhea, sometimes they get cured with home remedies, but sometimes they do not. They continue to be sick even if we take them to doctors. Sometimes they even die because of diarrhea.
—Kaqchikel Maya mother, Acatenango coffee plantation

A hush fell over Doña Flavia's patio in Panaj one afternoon as Rosario's fourteen-year-old daughter peeked around the gate and shyly called a greeting. She went over to where Flavia was weaving an intricately patterned *huipil* on her foot-pedal loom. After a short, whispered conversation, Flavia nodded and pointed the visitor over to the kitchen lean-to with her lips and a clicking sound that means, "Yep, over there." They went into the kitchen, the fire banked in a rare reprieve between meal preparation, and Flavia carefully scooped two big spoonfuls of sugar from a plastic bag into a cloth the girl pulled from her apron pocket. The girl twisted the cloth closed, murmured her thanks, and slipped away.

Flavia sat back down to continue her work while her adult daughter Maria, at her own loom, and I, crocheting misshapen hats to keep my hands busy, both looked up with questioning eyes. Flavia sighed. Rosario, who was still grieving baby Efraín, had a toddler with diarrhea. In Panaj, this was hardly remarkable. "It's to be expected," Flavia said, reflecting that the toddler had reached the age when diarrhea happens often. However, the loss of Efraín was a fresh reminder that something so common could turn deadly serious. Rosario was asking for some sugar to add to *atol*, a thin corn porridge, to give to the sick little one. Rosario did not have medicines in her home, but she was proud. She had sent a couple of precious 10-*centavo* coins over for the sugar, which Flavia shook her head at and refused. "We all do what we can," she said, "Rosario works hard, but she has too much to do. It's dirty over there, and those little ones always have a tail," using a colloquial term for having diarrhea. "They don't have a tap, and it's hard to get clean water," Flavia added.

Maria, a middle-aged mother of three young women who had lost her husband in the internal armed conflict, was not one to indulge in gossip and had been listening and nodding. She was quiet, thoughtful, and a meticulous homemaker. I admired her for her loving but no-nonsense attitude and felt lucky to have her watch my own two small children years later when I needed to attend meetings for work. But on the afternoon Rosario sent for sugar, she uncharacteristically chimed in with the scientific proclamation that, "there is no proven way to purify water." I could tell this statement was deeply felt, and I asked for clarification. "Well," Maria explained, "about two years ago, one group of gringos came and taught us that we could use empty plastic soda bottles up on the roof for a day to purify the water with the sun." At this point, Flavia broke in, "Water! Up on the roof! You see how tall we are! How would we reach up there all day?" Maria laughed. I could see her point. There is pervasive growth stunting among the Maya, and I tower over most adult women at my own modest five-foot-two-inch frame. Maria continued, "Then a year later, another group of gringos came and gave out bleach drops to put in the water. They say it works, but it tastes terrible." If you have ever swallowed swimming pool water, you will also know this is true. "Finally," Maria finished, "about six months ago a group from the health center came out, told us about hygiene again, and said we should boil our water. So, I think that it is all experiments, that there's no way to know for sure if water is clean."

Far more important than what microbiology could tell us about the untreated water sources in the community, Maria's statements, based on logic and reason applied to observed phenomena, told me an important story of water purification for Panaj. The struggles for clean water of families like Flavia's and Rosario's had not been resolved. The uncoordinated efforts of global health interventions, both foreign and government-sponsored programs, had led to confusion and a reasonable conclusion that there was no reliable way to purify water. I began asking around Panaj to see what others thought, and many agreed. I heard several reports of being satisfied with the intervention that promoted bleach, because they could use it for laundry and other cleaning. "It's our choice," a neighbor said, "they tell us things, but we decide [what we do]." Others talked about how much wood they would need if they were going to boil every mouthful of water they drank, which poses a huge burden either to cut wood from dwindling resources or to pay for it. I could easily imagine the one-sided zeal with which the three global health interventions were introduced into the community, enthusiasm for success blocking out conversation and the opportunity to learn about what had come before.

The messages on household water purification were confusing, with different options that each have their own implementation challenges. Similarly, different approaches to oral rehydration therapy (ORT) have introduced uncertainty. Three primary methods of oral rehydration education and distribution are employed in Rosario and Flavia's region in the Chimaltenango Department. First, for about forty years, government health facilities and nongovernmental organizations (NGOs) have distributed packets of oral rehydration salts (ORS) at no cost in rural communities, with instruction provided by local community health workers on the administration of ORT.[1] Second, branded packets of ORS and premixed bottled solution are available in pharmacies and even many small corner stores.[2] Third, a corporation sells oral rehydration solution as well as vitamins and other health supplements through a multilevel marketing scheme, using local representatives has gained a sizable market in Guatemala. Their marketing strategy relies on local vendors who sell the products to friends and relatives in their rural communities.

In this chapter, I explore the history of oral rehydration therapy as a key global health tool against severe outcomes from childhood diarrheal disease. This is essential to understand how global health programs and protocols, constructed in distant high-income countries, are introduced—and then actually experienced—in communities. I describe the traditional healing system common throughout Latin America and its contemporary role in Guatemala in relation to ORT. As we see in the case of water purification in Panaj, global health interventions often fall into the fallacy of the empty vessel, or the notion that they are the first to share relevant information in a community and that there are no existing deeply held beliefs and relevant experiences shaping interpretation of that information.[3] I also consider how cultural traditions and healing practices can be used to justify continued marginalization of Indigenous Maya populations from adequate health services. Finally, I discuss how the hygiene lessons that are commonplace in global water quality, sanitation, and hygiene (WASH) interventions can retrench stigma and racism. Throughout all the WASH interventions and ORT trainings in Panaj, the community had no choices on what they received. Global health organizations just showed up in their trucks and vans with information. Yet community members responded by choosing whether to engage, what to believe, and what to do in their own homes. As we will see, although global health programming positions communities as passive recipients, they are real people with agency who push back and shape how they engage with these programs.

The Development of ORT

Tragically, deaths like baby Efraín's happen every day in majority world countries where diarrhea remains a leading cause of death in children under the age of five and a major factor in undernutrition.[4] The effective treatment of diarrhea is an urgent and ever-present need across majority world countries and has been a focus of global health efforts for over sixty years. The development of ORT was a major public health breakthrough, enabling treatment of diarrhea within communities as never before possible. Though it seems simple to us now to focus on hydration, tackling treatment of diarrhea is a very complex problem. To start, diarrhea is not a singular disease entity but must be considered as a disease category. A vast range of pathogens can cause diarrhea, including bacteria, viruses, protozoa, and nematodes.[5] This makes treatment of diarrhea difficult because no one treatment will combat the underlying causal pathogen. Further, laboratory testing to discover the causal pathogen is cumbersome, requiring specialized equipment and skills, so it is not a practical approach to treating every case. The transmission of diarrheal agents also occurs in a variety of manners, including the direct fecal-oral route or through contaminated water supplies, so it can be difficult to identify and control sources of the sickness.

The nutritional consequences of diarrheal episodes are due to a number of factors, including food withholding, food refusal and vomiting during episodes, and the high costs of energy from the body that infections require. Reduced food consumption and poor absorption of nutrition in the gut leads to growth faltering during and after the diarrheal episode. The undernutrition that can result from diarrhea increases the likelihood of reinfection, perpetuating the disease cycle. We know that rural Maya children in Guatemala have high baseline rates of chronic undernutrition, meaning that their bodies are less prepared to fight and recover from diarrheal infections. Although early programs to control diarrheal disease focused on acute dehydrating diarrhea as responsible for the majority of deaths, we now recognize that many children who die have repeated episodes of diarrhea over a prolonged period and suffer profound undernutrition.[5] This was clearly the case for baby Efraín, who lost the fight with diarrhea and the drain of repeated infections on his tiny body. His death was resignedly ordinary in Panaj, where children in the village were often referred to as "having a tail" of diarrhea.

The persistent systemic challenges to improving baseline nutritional status in children have proved intractable despite twenty years of intensive government and NGO programs focusing on this issue in Guatemala.[7] Poor nutritional status goes a long way in explaining poor outcomes from diarrhea disease. This embodiment of poverty within rural Maya communities explains why my own round-cheeked boys have been fine following their few childhood experiences of diarrhea and Efraín and his siblings are put in mortal danger. ORT cannot fix the terrible systems of inequality that lead to these hard, corporeal facts. But ORT is a key life-saving strategy to prevent dehydration from diarrhea through the replacement of fluid and electrolytes. ORT simulates the composition of intestinal fluid lost in diarrhea, enabling the kidneys to continue to regulate the composition of body fluids. In addition to ORT, children with diarrhea should continue to be fed during a bout of diarrhea. Fluid and electrolyte losses can be counterbalanced by ORT, but it cannot provide all the adequate nutrition that an ill child requires.[8]

Before ORT was developed, intravenous (IV) therapy for dehydration caused by diarrhea was the standard of care established at the start of the twentieth century, and it is still used for severe cases. However, IV therapy has limitations, including the lack of availability of the equipment, supplies, and trained health staff needed to administer IV fluids safely in communities most affected in majority world countries.[9] The use of ORT in more severe cases became routine in the late 1960s, primarily in hospital settings and in refugee cholera outbreak situations.[10] The World Health Organization (WHO) adopted a standardized formula of ORT in 1975, updated in 2003 (see table 1.1).[11] WHO also initiated a global program to reduce diarrheal disease mortality in 1978, focused on moving ORT out of tertiary care settings and into communities.[12]

Table 1.1
WHO-recommended ingredients of oral rehydration salts.

Ingredient	Amount (grams/liter)
Glucose	13.5
Sodium chloride	2.6
Trisodium citrate dihydrate	2.9
Potassium chloride	1.5

Source: World Health Organization. 2006. Oral rehydration salts: Production of the new solution. https://www.who.int/publications/i/item/WHO-FCH-CAH-06.1.

UNICEF, WHO, USAID, and other donors have undertaken a massive worldwide program to provide ORS to children in low-resource settings. This strategy emerged in the 1960s and continues to be a cornerstone of global health delivery.[13] Throughout the late 1970s and 1980s, WHO and UNICEF led campaigns for the distribution of ORT and the implementation of diarrhea control programs in most countries worldwide.[14] ORT was touted as a breakthrough "simple solution" for treating one of the most intractable global health problems since it requires no special equipment, technical skills, or complex supply chain.[15] The focus of global health programs addressing diarrhea shifted from clinical settings to education on the use of ORT for child caregivers and community health workers, community members trained to serve as the frontline of primary health care. In Guatemala, UNICEF took a key role in providing ORS packets in collaboration with the Ministry of Health, and the Pan American Health Organization, the regional office of the WHO, provided technical assistance and training for health workers. The Nutrition Institute of Central America and Panama (INCAP, for its acronym in Spanish) provided technical assistance throughout the region and conducted critical longitudinal studies of child nutritional status and growth in Guatemala, where the institute is based.[16]

In 1992, WHO estimated 73 percent of people across the globe had access to ORS and that oral rehydration therapy was used in 38 percent of all diarrheal cases. WHO also found that four out of five packets of oral rehydration salts were produced in the country where they were used in 1992, marking an important shift toward decreased reliance on the global health structures that initiated ORT programs. Efforts to spread ORT had reduced child deaths from dehydration by over one million per annum.[17]

Since the time of the adoption of the standard ORT formula by the WHO in 1975, ongoing clinical research has sought to optimize its safety and efficacy in the treatment and prevention of dehydration in diarrhea, resulting in a (slightly) updated standard formula in 2003.[18]

In 1980, an estimated one billion episodes of diarrheal disease resulted in 4.6 million deaths annually in children under five years of age, occurring primarily in Africa, Asia, and Latin America.[19] The figures ten years later indicated that there was a changing pattern in mortality, with rates dropping to 3.3 million deaths per year, but the incidence of infection remained largely unchanged from the figures of 1980.[20] More recent estimates show a significant reduction in deaths to 525,000 annually in children under five, yet morbidity remains high at an estimated 1.7 billion cases of childhood diarrhea.[21] This reduction in mortality is largely attributed to improvements in management of diarrheal disease, mainly through the introduction of oral rehydration therapy to prevent death from dehydration. These successes stem from sustained global health programming efforts related to ORT, led by WHO technical experts and implementation guidelines, while efforts to reduce incidence of childhood diarrheal disease through improved water and sanitation systems have seen more muted success. Despite the exciting successes of ORT, diarrhea remains a leading cause of death of children globally, and reductions in morbidity and mortality have been unevenly distributed in low-resource contexts.[22]

Implementation of ORT

While the clinical efficacy of ORT is clear, it can only impact childhood diarrheal disease outcomes if concerted efforts are made by health systems to support community use and in-community training.[23] The challenge of getting ORT to every child in villages like Panaj across Guatemala and throughout the majority world is complex. In global health, implementation is everything. WHO campaigns promoting ORT have included primarily the dissemination of ORS packets. Yet the overreliance on packaged ORS in the preliminary global push for ORT coverage may have limited the enduring success of ORT educational efforts. While clinical research energies have been focused on maximizing the benefits of the standard ORS formula, less consistent attention has been given to education about how to effectively give ORT to a child and the use of homemade solutions. The efficacy of household fluids and foods in preventing and treating diarrhea-related dehydration has been well established, but homemade approaches have been supported in fits and starts by WHO and UNICEF ORT programs.[24]

In the example of ORT, we see a core challenge to global health structures and systems. Shared technical expertise, program manuals, and toolkits are a critical resource for majority world countries that may have limited internal capacity to develop such tools, but their benefits are leavened by the homogenizing nature of universal guidelines. They are simply not able to account for the relevant assets and needs that local delivery contexts have. There are often prompts in WHO guidelines to adapt to the local context, but for the very reasons countries need external assistance on required supplies, systems, and expertise, majority world countries are often unable to do meaningful work to adapt guidelines to their unique circumstances. National governments are positioned as recipients and have little choice in shaping the global health guidance and programs they get. There are always benefits and burdens.

WHO guidelines on the management of diarrheal disease and treatment protocols provide a framework for how ORT can be integrated into a system of care from the community level to facility-based care for severe cases.[25] These guidelines have been adopted in the Guatemalan government health system, where all health providers from clinicians to nurses to community health workers are instructed in the Ministry of Health's treatment plan for diarrhea based on WHO recommendations (see table 1.2). The goal of the protocol is to enable health staff to quickly triage children with diarrhea for severity and to treat them appropriately or refer severe cases for a higher level of care.

Under the WHO guidelines, ORT may be administered through a variety of methods, including homemade solutions. Currently, the primary national ORT program in Guatemala is through the delivery of free packets of ORS, manufactured in-country, to caregivers of children on an as-needed basis through health centers and mobile health teams. While this may be the most effective means of maximizing efficacy, water must still be added in the appropriate quantity, and the cost of the packaging drastically raises the cost of a dose of ORS. Further, it is unrealistic to imagine that packaged ORS can be provided to every child with a case of diarrhea. At a societal level, the reliance on packaged solutions can entrench health system access issues between patients and health providers; at a global health

Table 1.2

Guatemalan Ministry of Health treatment plan for children with diarrhea.

	Plan A	Plan B	Plan C
Definition	Light	Moderate	Grave
Loss of body fluid	Less than 5% body weight	6–9% body weight	More than 10% body weight
General condition	Normal, alert	Irritable	Lethargic, unconscious
Eyes	Normal, with tears	Sunken, no tears	Very sunken, dry
Tongue/oral membranes	Wet	Dry	Very dry
Thirst	Drinking normally	Drinking avidly, thirsty	Drinking little or unable to drink
Skin pliability	Retracts normally	Retracts in less than 2 seconds	Retracts in more than 2 seconds
Decision	No signs of dehydration	If more than 2 Plan B signs, clinical dehydration	If more than 2 Plan C signs, severe dehydration
Treatment	• Give ORT after each diarrhea • Do not withhold food, fluids	• Give 50–100 cc of ORT per kg of weight at rate of 1/4 total solution per hour • If vomiting, consider Plan C	• Use when Plan B does not work • Begin IV fluid • Refer to nearest inpatient facility

Source: Morales, M. S. 2004. *Informe Final de Investigación Epidemiológica: Factores de Riesgo Asociados a Morbilidad por Diarrea en Niños de Cinco Años de San Juan Comalapa, Chimaltenango.* Universidad de San Carlos de Guatemala.

systems level, it can perpetuate a giver–receiver power dynamic between countries.[26]

Over the last fifteen years, I have heard a lot of stories about previous ORT campaigns. When I tell people I am interested in treatments for childhood diarrheal disease, I tend to get giggles and then the stories start coming. I have heard stories about an NGO that distributed special sets of spoons designed to measure sugar and salt in the WHO-recommended amounts for mixing with water. Other strategies have included the pinch/scoop method, where a pinch of salt and a scoop of sugar are added to water to make ORS at home. In Chimaltenango, several NGOs had adopted this approach in the 1970s and 1980s, using a 12-ounce glass Coke bottle with a pinch of salt, adding a scoop of sugar using the metal lid, and then filling the bottle with water up to the top of the logo. I heard stories about these efforts from older women, but I never saw anyone use these strategies in communities.

Trends in the use of home fluids in ORT have mirrored broader trends in global health. When global health has favored highly focused programs for disease eradication, it has also favored packaged ORS. When global health has focused on primary care and health systems strengthening, ORT efforts have included training caregivers in the preparation and administration of home oral rehydration solutions. Recommended home fluids include soup, rice water, yogurt drinks, and plain water.[27] Prevailing wisdom during the 1980s and 1990s, a period of global health emphasizing primary care, held that only households experiencing severe famine would lack the necessary ingredients to make a sufficient solution for oral rehydration therapy and that only knowledge is lacking.[28] Though homemade solutions may be variable in their nutrient, electrolyte, and fluid content, they have been shown to be effective in preventing dehydration from diarrhea. Homemade ORS solutions have been made a part of the educational component of some recent ORT campaigns again, including encouraging specific recipes using widely available local ingredients. The cost and inconvenience of needing to get packaged ORS outside the home is a barrier to ORT use that home fluids can help address.[29] Across various types of ORT programs, implementation strategies have focused on the education of caregivers, primarily mothers, on how and when to administer the promoted form of ORT.[30]

Limitations of ORT

A key limitation of the ORT strategy is that it does not address the causes or reduce incidence rates of diarrheal disease. Only improved water supplies and sanitation systems can do that. The Millennium Development Goals, the targets set at the turn of the millennium by United Nations member states to improve specific global health and development targets by 2015, and their continuation through the 2030 Sustainable Development Goals, have made important advancements in improved water sources and sanitation.[31] Although it fell short on most of the goals, Guatemala was heralded as a huge success on Millennium Development Goal 7c: Access to Improved Water Supply, with total population access estimated to have increased from a baseline of 77 percent in 1990 to 91 percent by the target year for the goals in 2015.[32] While there continued to be urban and rural disparities in the reach of access to improved water supplies, there were exciting gains in the expansion of municipal water systems and piped water into households and shared communal spaces.[33] Children in Guatemala who have access to treated piped water have lower incidence of diarrhea.[34] However, maintenance of community-level water treatment systems has proven to be challenging due to low political will and poor infrastructural and institutional development, so household-level water purification remains important in preventing diarrhea.[35] Only US$1.3 million was allocated for water quality efforts in the Ministry of Health budget for 2017, indicating a strong reliance on foreign aid in this sector.[36] As a result, Guatemala has struggled to make sustained progress on the Sustainable Development Goals related to water and sanitation.

In Panaj, an open-air lagoon provides water for much of the community, but the pump house fell into disrepair, and the village council has struggled to keep the water flowing (see figure 1.1). When water came through the pipes to Flavia's house, it had not been treated with the chemicals required

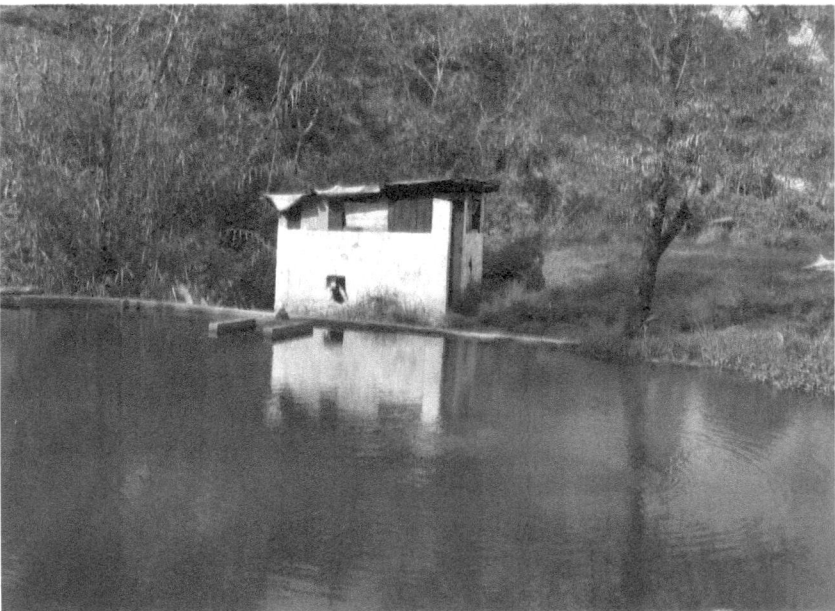

Figure 1.1
Lagoon and pump house in Panaj.

to ensure it would be free of diarrheal pathogens. Much fanfare was made of the modern convenience and cleanliness of the piped water supplies. To be sure, the women and girls of Panaj enjoyed not needing to walk down to the lagoon or to one of the local springs to carry water home. But they did not know that the convenience of water piped into or nearby their homes could be carrying invisible diarrheal pathogens—a trick of development that feels like two steps forward, one step backward. The stopgap measure of oral rehydration would no longer be so acutely necessary if the promise of the Millennium Development Goals' success was being lived in communities.

I have often observed ORT trainings both for community health workers and caregivers where the trainer, in an attempt to encourage ORT use, has said it will stop the diarrhea. ORT does not stop diarrhea—it is not intended to do that. One of the challenges of community-based education on ORT use is that it can be incredibly counterintuitive: when a child is well hydrated during diarrhea, more liquid feces is produced. It is a good sign that they continue to be hydrated, but the high volume of diarrhea can be concerning for caregivers—it is alarming to feel that you are making a child's diarrhea worse. As a result, caregivers sometimes withhold food and liquids from children during an episode of diarrhea.[37] In 2004, WHO updated the recommendations for ORT to include the coadministration of zinc supplementation.[38] The benefits of the addition of zinc supplementation alongside ORT are that it helps shorten the bout of diarrhea and can help prevent reinfection for one month following administration.[39] Zinc was adopted in the Guatemalan national formulary for this purpose in 2011, and funding for 4 million doses was announced.[40]

A study in Guatemala found that co-packaging of ORS and zinc made health providers more likely to give both ORS and zinc and for caregivers to administer both to children with diarrhea.[41] The same project also found that child caregivers perceived greater value in treating diarrhea when ORS and zinc were co-packaged.[42] Unfortunately, the collaboration with the Canadian government that supported this project ended, and it was not taken on by the Guatemalan Ministry of Health. Both ORT and zinc are now the first-line treatment protocol for child diarrhea, but access challenges persist. An exciting short-term project funded through foreign aid pointed to an evidence-based best practice to improve uptake and administration of

ORT, but the funding could not be maintained by the Guatemalan health system. So nothing happened.

Similarly, I was part of a study team that investigated community use of ORT and zinc after training with community health workers in a rural Guatemalan town. The training emphasized good home fluids to administer in ORT. Use of ORT increased, and preferred ORS changed from packaged to homemade solutions during the study. However, the use of zinc did not change at all—because there was never any zinc available in the community health post for the entirety of the two-year study period.[43] In fact, the government health worker assigned to the local health post became annoyed when community members asserted their knowledge of zinc and demanded it for their sick children, only to be told that there was none. The reality within the community did not match the protocols on paper or the promises of department level health officials that zinc was widely available and free for patients. In this case, a regional Ministry of Health official turned out to be diverting the zinc supplies received from the central government stockpile for private, for-profit sale.

Although zinc, when available, can mitigate one of the challenges of promoting ORT by shortening the duration of diarrhea, some further challenges remain to this no-so-simple solution. Time to administer ORT can be laborious, requiring that a spoonful be given as often as every fifteen minutes.[44] For caregivers, who are almost exclusively women and girls (as we will see further in chapter 2), this can create an unmanageable burden when there may be other children who require care, household tasks, and income-generating labor that must also be completed. I have sat in many trainings, and even given some myself, knowing that the ideal guidance of slow and steady administration of ORT could not be achieved in the reality of daily life for Guatemalan mothers.

While zinc can help prevent a subsequent bout of diarrhea for about a month, children in Guatemala face constant exposure to diarrheal pathogens because of the lack of clean water and sanitation systems. Children experience an average of one bout of diarrhea each month in Guatemala.[45] For a population experiencing ongoing food insecurity, particularly among the 70 percent of the Mayan population who cannot meet their nutritional needs and are chronically undernourished, this can have lifelong impacts.[46] Children's bodies must use up precious calories fighting off infection after infection, which is energy diverted from growth.[47] Fifty percent of all Indigenous Maya children in Guatemala experience growth stunting, the highest rates in the Western hemisphere and the fourth highest in the world.[48] Until recently, the Guatemalan government relied on notions that Maya populations were genetically short in stature rather than acknowledge the reality that their shortness (even shorter than at the time of conquest 500 years ago) is a biosocial marker of structural inequality.[49]

Though ORT programs have a long history in the Chimaltenango Department, coverage has not been complete and successes equivocal. While a very high proportion of mothers reported having heard of ORT, few had ever tried to use it.[50] My long-term ethnographic data indicate that very few caregivers use ORT regularly. As Rosario's request to borrow sugar from Flavia shows, packets of ORT or even the ingredients to make a simple homemade solution are not always on hand. Many Maya caregivers in rural, poor communities do not use ORT regularly, or if they do, they use it in combination with other pharmaceuticals or traditional treatments. Syncretism, or incorporation of biomedical knowledge into humoral belief systems and traditional healing practices, has occurred widely in Guatemala and throughout Latin America. The syncretism of traditional healing practices and ORT opens up a wide range of choices that caregivers must navigate. It can be both empowering to blend and choose what works for their families and potentially overwhelming to know what the right choices are and try to access them. We cannot fully understand the choices Rosario made in navigating health-seeking options for baby Efraín without situating them within this broader health care landscape.

Traditional Healing and Medical Pluralism in Guatemala

The first time I met Doña Merilda, I knocked nervously on her corrugated tin door. She was a neighbor of the family I lived with in Comalapa, and when they heard that I wanted to learn about treatments for childhood diarrhea, they sent me straight to her. After what seemed like a long wait with the guys in the shop across the street staring at me, the door creaked slowly open. The curious look in Doña Merilda's eyes was quickly replaced by a smile on her face—the unusual event of a *gringa* showing up on her doorstep did not seem to faze her. She had heard from her neighbors about me. I was getting famous! For diarrhea! She invited me into her home's long patio that runs the length of the house and is filled with plants that she uses for her remedies. Doña Merilda is a fifty-nine-year-old Kaqchikel Maya woman, a healer and trusted source of advice in her community. Over many years, she has become a mentor and friend. She patiently describes her treatments and clucks her tongue in gentle rebuke when I (always) forget the names of plants, and she (always) asks why I am a bit fatter or thinner than the last time I saw her. She misses nothing.

Doña Merilda's working conception of body structure and function holds that the stomach is surrounded at all times by a sac that holds worms. A humorally balanced diet and body temperature typically keep the worms satiated and content inside their sac, but upsets in the body's balance can cause the worms to become agitated and leave the sac. This results in worm-induced diarrhea, including the condition *empacho*, an illness characterized by a swollen stomach, painful cramping, and gas. Cases of diarrhea attributed to worms are much more common in children, whose bodily balance is far more delicate than adults.

Doña Merilda regularly mixes biomedical treatments and Catholic prayers with her more traditional treatments. She is like many other practicing "traditional" healers in her syncretism of elements of traditional healing and popular home remedies. She picks and chooses from the treatments known to her based on personal experience of efficacy. She often tells mothers to buy a particular biomedical remedy from a pharmacy, such as Alka-Seltzer or acetaminophen, to use in conjunction with her treatments for their children. Doña Merilda also frequently recommends that her child patients be taken to the health center if she perceives that the sickness is severe and that she will not be able to treat it successfully. In the same vein, she noted that she also has patients who come to her after an unsatisfactory visit to the health center. Healers like Doña Merilda are "traditional" in that they support local cultural norms and preferences in care-seeking. Though there is a charge for service, and Doña Merilda earns a living by caring for her community, the charges are flexible and based on the mutuality of community relationships. Doña Merilda is not, however, a throwback to another time, often imagined as simpler and purer in its expression of Maya culture. She is a contemporary practitioner who uses all of the tools at her disposal to care for her patients.

Though I never heard Doña Merilda recommend purchasing ORT to a mother, she told me that she thinks ORT is very useful for children with diarrhea. She said, "*Suero oral* [ORT] is good because it keeps the kids hydrated [and] their eyes moist. It is good for diarrhea." Unlike in many of my interviews with local mothers, Doña Merilda recognized that ORT does not cure diarrhea but that its key benefit is in keeping children hydrated. I persistently asked her on multiple occasions how she would differentiate the types of diarrhea for which ORT would be useful, and she consistently answered that ORT is good for all types of diarrhea. I asked specifically about her distinctions between treatments for hot, cold, and worm-induced diarrheas, and she held fast to her assertion that ORT would be useful in each of these categories. This contradicts previous research findings that traditional humoral systems in Latin America would prevent the use of ORT for some categories of diarrhea, such as empacho.[51]

Health-seeking behaviors take place across different interacting systems and sets of beliefs, including the traditional, popular, and biomedical sectors.[52] The relationships among health sectors within a society may be based on cooperation or competition. In Guatemala, as in most societies, the biomedical sector has become dominant, yet the traditional and popular sectors remain central to contemporary health beliefs and practices, as we see in Doña Merilda's practice. The traditional sector has a significant presence in most Latin American countries, with variations on specific form by country and region.[53]

Guatemala has an incredibly pluralistic health care landscape across which individual patients and their families must navigate the range of choices dictated by cost and accessibility.[54] The Guatemalan government health system and the philanthropic and private sectors each contribute to this pluralism— the coexistence of different healing approaches, treatments, and institutions that care-seekers choose among. We must understand the traditional Indigenous healing system and its current practice in order to contextualize the use of ORT in Guatemala. Many Indigenous systems of healing in Latin America are rooted in humoral beliefs about the body, where health in part depends on the maintenance of a delicate balance of bodily elements, including hot and cold. Within the Latin American region, many early ORT campaigns failed to consider the salience of long-held humoral beliefs and promoted ORT in a way that was inconsistent with those beliefs.

Europeans brought humoral medical beliefs to the Americas during conquest and colonization, though sophisticated medical systems were already in place in many areas before the arrival of Europeans. In fact, Hernando

Cortés was apparently so impressed by the herbal knowledge and therapies he encountered in Mexico that he felt bringing Spanish doctors to the New World was unnecessary.[55] The humoral theory of Spanish physicians was overlaid on existing Indigenous healing practices and attributed most disease causality to natural rather than supernatural causes. George Foster asserted that acceptance of humoral theory in post-Columbian Latin America was widespread because it provided a simple framework that could encompass the internal logic and practices within both Spanish and Indigenous American traditions.[56] Further, Indigenous American cosmologies at the time of Spanish conquest were based on binary classificatory relationships; this melded well with humoral theory, which is based on the hot and cold binary.[57]

Although there is great variation in humoral medical systems across Latin America, some key features are shared. First, two types of temperature affect the human system: thermal temperature, which can be measured, and metaphoric temperature, which characterizes all food and remedies. Second, a healthy human body temperature should err slightly toward the "hot" end of the hot-cold temperature spectrum. Third, the body's temperature equilibrium is upset when the body is exposed to either thermal or metaphoric cold or heat. Heating experiences include digestion of food, sleeping, emotional experiences, pregnancy, ingestion of metaphorically Hot food and drink, and external exposure to metaphorically Hot materials.[58] Likewise, cooling experiences include loss of warm blood from menstruation, childbirth, or surgery; thermal chills from exposure to cold air or water; and ingestion of thermally or metaphorically Cold food and drink. Finally, a body in a heated state, either thermally or metaphorically, is at risk of illness from additional exposure to either hot or cold influences. For example, sleeping warms the body but does not in itself cause illness. Yet, if someone who has just awoken bathes, drinks cold water, or is exposed to any other cold influences, they can expect to be affected by a range of possible ailments, including bronchitis, toothaches, and headaches.[59]

"Traditional" Mayan healing, of which the humoral system came to form an important part, has continued to evolve since the time of conquest and colonization. It coexists and intertwines across the popular and biomedical health sectors. The latter half of the twentieth century was marked by the increased expansion and importance of biomedicine in Latin America, and a rich period of study of medical pluralism and syncretism occurred at the turn of the century. Indigenous taxonomies for illnesses in Guatemala, including diarrhea, show change over time.[60] The syncretism of biomedical and humoral beliefs incorporates accessible elements of biomedicine with existing humoral beliefs about causality and treatment. This syncretism is well illustrated in a key study of beliefs about childhood diarrhea in rural Guatemala.[61] Diarrhea, generally known as *asientos*, is a well-recognized illness, although it is sometimes classified as merely a symptom of other diseases. Diarrhea in Guatemala and much of Latin America may also be seen as related to milestones in a child's growth, such as teething, crawling, and walking. This illustrates the ubiquity of childhood diarrhea to the degree that it is often seen as an inevitable component of the growth process. Diarrhea is not recognized as an illness when it occurs in conjunction with particular developmental milestones.[62]

Prior research has found two primary explanatory models for diarrhea in the rural Guatemalan villages. The first was, as described above, the belief that an inappropriate balance of either thermally or metaphorically Hot and Cold foods had been ingested, resulting in the imbalance of body temperature and diarrhea, a thermally hot illness.[63] As in Doña Merilda's practice, the second causal belief about diarrhea concerned the idea that worms function in the normal process of digestion in a sac in the abdomen. An improper humoral balance of foods ingested can disturb the worms, and they can leave their sac to travel through the body and cause potentially fatal diarrheal illness. Interestingly, this prior research found that, in conjunction with traditional humoral explanations of diarrhea, many informants also implicated lack of hygiene, consistent with biomedical explanations for the transmission of diarrheal pathogens, as causes of diarrhea. The authors explain:

> As many medical anthropologists have noted in the past, the cluster of explanations related to cold, worms and eating reflects underlying beliefs about physiology which are sharply different from those of the biomedical perspective. *Dirtiness as a cause, however, is much closer to the biomedical notion of the transmission of pathogens through faecal-oral contamination, even though the specific mechanisms by which women believe dirtiness causes diarrhea may be quite different.*[64]

Perhaps the incorporation of ideas of "dirtiness" into the Indigenous etiology of diarrhea can be attributed to the binary nature of the humoral system and the biomedical categorization of dirt.[65] It also indicates an onboarding of global health hygiene messages.

Some medical anthropologists have suggested that the dominant influence of biomedicine has shifted the primary importance of humoral medicine to instances of self-diagnosis, where individuals or parents and caretakers of children assess the cause of an illness in order to select an appropriate course of treatment.[66] However, others believe that the role of traditional humoral medicine may be experiencing resurgence even in urban areas of Latin America, perhaps due to lack of accessibility of biomedical care.[67] As part of this resurgence, Maya traditional healing practices are sometimes romanticized by those outside of Maya communities—*ladinos* looking for a cure and eager anthropologists are both guilty parties. Humoral practices can have negative health impacts, such as through dietary restrictions placed on pregnant and postpartum women and sick children. For example, many women avoid cooling foods after childbirth because the loss of Hot blood during delivery means they must have warming foods to rebalance. Further, humoral beliefs can affect the uptake of some biomedical treatments, mostly considered metaphorically Hot, though I have not seen this to be the case for ORT or other medicines used for treatment of diarrhea.[68]

ORT and Traditional Healing

An example from Honduras in the early 1980s illustrates how differences in Indigenous and biomedical beliefs about causes and treatments of diarrhea can lead to the failure of an ORT intervention. In this study, residents of a village in that country were asked to identify the causes they associated with the symptoms of diarrhea. They responded with four main causes: *empacho, ojo* (evil eye), *caida de mollera* (fallen fontanelles), and *lombrices* (worms). In the village, use of ORT tied to a government-planned intervention was high for all causes of diarrheal symptoms except for *empacho*. Empacho is a painful blockage of the gut brought on by eating the wrong types of food, the wrong combination of foods on the Hot–Cold scale, eating at improper times, or eating foods that are incompletely cooked. Traditional healers treat empacho by massaging the body and administering a purgative to clear the system of its "dirty" contents.[69]

After two years, the study found that, as anticipated, usage of ORT for episodes of empacho remained low. The authors attribute this to differences of belief: if empacho requires a purgative, then ORT would not satisfy those requirements within the Indigenous humoral system. The government organizers of the campaign were unwilling to market ORT as a purgative in order to make it acceptable within the medical system of the targeted population. In this instance, the ORT campaign was essentially asking the population to reverse their beliefs about the functioning of the body in order to accept the biomedical ideas of the ORT campaign.[70] The project did not collaborate with the local population but rather worked against prevailing ideas of diarrheal diagnosis and treatment. Hence, taking into account the prevalent medical system and health-seeking behaviors for diarrhea is crucial to the efficacy of ORT campaigns in Latin America so that campaigns may be structured in a way that is as compatible as possible with existing ideas and treatments.

In working on ORT programs in Guatemala, I have witnessed this incompatibility of ideas firsthand, but it does not have to remain a barrier to care. A few years ago, I was helping prepare materials for a community ORT training program in which local women trained as community health promoters. They, in turn, trained their peers on the use of ORT and diarrhea danger signs. Rice water, plantain water, and especially maize water are all options for liquids to make ORT, and all were available in villages. Given the omnipresent pot of ground maize available to make porridge and the dietary staple of tortillas in most homes, maize water made particular sense as a choice. To make ORT, you only need to skim off some of the cloudy water while boiling rice, plantains, or maize; this starchy water has an appropriate balance of electrolytes to act as ORT. A few of the other suggestions, such as yogurt drinks and premixed ORS, were seen as appealing by the community health promoters but less likely to be used in the community because of their cost and availability. However, chicken broth, widely available and consumed regularly, was outright rejected by the community health promoters as an option for homemade ORT. My North American health provider colleague began to argue with the promoters, pointing out the benefits and availability of chicken broth. The community health promoters would not say why they would not use chicken broth, only that no one ever would. When I quietly told my colleague that it would be heating for an already Hot condition, the women smiled with relief. There were plenty of other good and available solutions, and it only took listening to discover what would mesh with local preferences and humoral beliefs.

Across the years of my work on child health and diarrheal disease in Guatemala, women have occasionally raised the concept of diarrhea being caused by humoral imbalances and discussed the home remedies they would use for such cases. I completed two series of focus-group discussions designed to draw out understanding of diarrhea and preferred local treatments.[71] During a focus group discussion, one woman said, to the nods and agreement of the entire group, "When it [diarrhea] is caused by heat it is yellow, but when it is already an infection, they defecate mucus sometimes. When this is the case, we use fresh herbs, rice flour, or citrus juice." Color of the stool has been shown to be the primary mechanism for determining the hot or cold nature of a bout of diarrhea in previous studies of Indigenous classification of diarrhea in Guatemala.[72]

In nearly all instances where people brought up humoral imbalance, herbs featured prominently in home treatments. Many of the herbal treatments mentioned reflect previous anthropological research on Maya classification and treatment of diarrhea in Guatemala.[73] Herbs are used to soothe the stomach, and they are used differently according to the hot or cold classification of the case of diarrhea. Diarrhea caused by heat is more likely to be treated with green herbs being placed on the outside of the body. However, diarrhea caused by cold (and more common during the cold months) is more often treated with teas created by boiling the herbs with water. The primary exception that I found to these general strategies of herbal home remedies was in cases where diarrhea was believed to be caused by worms. Different measures, usually involving the application of an external poultice to calm the worms, are taken for these types of diarrhea, and the help of a local healer is typically sought.

In my research, humoral classification of diarrhea and of appropriate herbal treatments did not affect women's likelihood of using ORT. When asked if ORT was good for some types of diarrhea but not for other types, women respond that it is good for all types, except when worms were implicated and additional measures to placate the worms would be necessary. As one mother in Acatenango explained, "Yes, *suero oral* (ORT) works for both types of diarrhea because when it is caused by heat, it refreshes their stomach, and when it is caused by cold, it helps them not get dehydrated."

Therefore, even when mothers do explain or categorize diarrhea in humoral terms as hot or cold, this categorization did not necessarily change their likelihood of ORT use. This finding is in contrast to previous studies of ORT in Latin America, including the study of empacho in Mexico, which indicated that the humoral system would prevent the use of ORT for some Indigenous classifications of diarrhea.[74]

Syncretism of herbal remedies and packaged medicines is common. Though the humoral system may shape some choices, such as the refusal of chicken broth as an ORS solution, use of this system does not correlate with the refusal of biomedical care. Traditional humoral and biomedical systems are inextricably intertwined—not mutually exclusive—in contemporary Guatemala.[75] No mother I have spoken with over the past fifteen years has said that she would forgo biomedical treatment in favor of traditional healing methods for a case of diarrhea that was deemed serious. However, facile and monolithic notions of "the Maya" continue to shape health system decisions in Guatemala, potentially aided and abetted by now-outdated anthropological research showing that the humoral system affected engagement with biomedical care. Once several years ago, when I was sitting in on a Ministry of Health meeting for the Chimaltenango Department, I heard the director for the region and his staff voice frustration at poor attendance at the rural health posts for primary care. He shook his head dismissively and said they could not do anything more than what they were doing. After the meeting was over, I asked him to explain. He sucked his teeth and jangled the change in his pocket and said, "They [Maya communities] don't really want our health care. They have their own beliefs, and they use their own healers." My heart sank for Rosario and Flavia and care-seekers throughout Maya communities. Through this cultural violence, Maya culture is used against Maya communities to deny the right to accessible health care.

ORT in Contemporary Guatemala

Despite encouraging statistics on coverage of ORT campaigns in Latin America and decreases in diarrheal morbidity and mortality, the successes of ORT campaigns in the region and in Guatemala have faced challenges. It is nearly impossible to measure ORT use rates since most cases of diarrhea are treated in the home; beyond that, it is hard to measure if ORT is being given correctly when it is used. For example, a meta-study of seventy-six surveys of

ORT use in thirty-six countries showed that an encouraging 58 percent of households used an ORS solution or a recommended home solution. Yet, only 32 percent of those households actually increased the amount of fluid given to the child experiencing diarrhea, and only 20.5 percent actually both increased fluids and continued feeding. Therefore, only about one in five children who were reported as receiving ORT actually received an effective application of ORT.[76] Therefore, the figures for ORT usage in Latin America are likely to overrepresent the actual numbers of households effectively using ORT. Further, national governments in Latin America may have incentives for inflating the amount of ORT promotion that they have done to meet funding guidelines for global health programs supported by foreign aid.[77]

The preference of government health systems in the majority world, including the Guatemalan Ministry of Health, for packaged ORS has led to economic dependencies and the inaccessibility of ORT for many. ORS packets are low cost and easy to store, and—perhaps most importantly in contemporary neoliberal global health—they are easy to count. Childhood diarrheal disease defies efforts toward metrics and accurate case-counts, but ORS packets give us something to count. The number of ORS packets distributed give us a metric of success. What gets counted in neoliberal global health gets funded. Yet, coverage of ORT remains below 50 percent in most countries, and an estimated 6.5 million cases of child diarrhea were not treated with any form of ORT in 2017.[78]

Promotion of ORS packets at the national level leads to dependence on foreign aid, and even if packets are produced in-country, unequal distribution of packets within countries can maintain and entrench regional inequalities. Guatemala was one of only a few countries where in-country inequality of ORT coverage actually increased between 2000 and 2017.[79] This reflects the broad trend in Latin America that poverty continues to be most concentrated in rural areas. Data from Guatemala show that 63 percent of rural residents live in poverty in comparison to 34 percent of urban residents.[80] When ORS packets are produced in-country, they remain more easily obtained by the wealthier urban populations to the detriment of rural ones. A fixed schedule of distribution to remote rural areas may be difficult if not impossible and does not solve challenges with seepage from the supply chain due to damage and corruption, making ORS scarce and oftentimes expensive for rural residents, as we saw in the case of zinc supplementation. The unnecessary dependency of rural communities on packaged ORS solutions has resulted in instances of diarrhea mortality where no packets were available and, as a result, no ORT was administered to the ill child.[81]

Although UNICEF no longer actively contributes to the day-to-day distribution of ORT in Guatemala, it maintains an in-country stockpile of ORS packets to be used in national emergencies and disaster relief, such as in the aftermath of Hurricane Stan in 2005 and Tropical Storm Agatha in 2010. Several NGOs in Guatemala also work on ORT and take a variety of approaches, from distributing ORS packets to providing education on how to make at-home ORS solutions. I had assumed that the long history of ORT programming in the Chimaltenango Department would have a cumulative effect, with knowledge building over time and across generations. Over the fifteen years that I have been asking questions about ORT in the Guatemalan highlands, the number of people who say that they have heard of ORT has grown. However, I have not found increases of knowledge on how to use ORT. I know from health care workers that ORT trainings are more sporadic than systematic and depend on what has captured the interest of government campaigns and foreign donors. A cumulative change can only happen if ORT education and promotion is consistent.

Premixed, bottled forms of ORT are by far the type of ORT most favored in Chimaltenango. Mothers say that their children prefer them to anything else because they taste so much better than powdered packets. Mothers reported that children like to have different flavors, and the bright colors are nice. By far, ladino mothers living in town in Chimaltenango said that they tend to buy bottled ORT at pharmacies if they try to give ORT to their children. For mothers out in the smaller towns of Acatenango and Comalapa, bottled solutions were also the preferred form of ORT. Yet, both ladino and Indigenous mothers cannot always afford bottled solutions, in which case they use packets from a pharmacy or health center if they decide to use ORT. Overall, the number of mothers making homemade ORT is very low. Only about one percent of both Indigenous and ladino women reported that they would make ORT in their home.[82] However, Indigenous women living in rural settings are more likely to use homemade solutions. Women who have tried rice water as an ORS solution report that it does not work because children will not drink it because it seems very unappealing. When directly asked whether homemade ORT or ORS packets are better, one mother said, "The ones in the packets are better because they are actually from the doctor. They work better. But kids don't like any of it because it tastes salty."

When considering the gradation of urban to rural and relative wealth to poverty, elements of social status associated with the different types of ORT begin to emerge. A lower middle-class to middle-class ladino mother would not think of going to a health center or post to acquire free packets of ORT. Such women would go to a private pharmacy to buy bottled solution or, at the very least, buy their own powdered packets. Conversely, rural Indigenous mothers who do not have the money to purchase bottled solutions rely on free or low-cost sources of packets or homemade ORS solutions.

Another significant element of safely administering ORT is knowing when to discard leftover solution. ORS solution should be thrown away twenty-four hours after it has been mixed. The paucity of free packets available from health posts and community health workers or the high cost of purchased solutions would make discarding something valuable counterintuitive for families who are accustomed to wasting nothing. Having a bottle of manufactured ORS solution becomes a status symbol, a sign of both affluence and of what might be interpreted as scrupulous care for one's child. This was, of course, not an option for Rosario as she sent her daughter to borrow a scoop of sugar from Flavia's kitchen to make homemade ORS.

The Stigma of Hygiene

I was spending time traveling with a mobile team outside of Comalapa, which included health care workers who visited rural communities on a monthly schedule to provide primary care, prenatal and pediatric growth checks, vaccinations, and basic medicines. One day as we entered the courtyard of a rural home, one of the nurses, herself from a rural Kaqchikel background, leaned over to me and said, "Look how dirty they are." I looked up, shocked, and she shook her head and tsk-tsked as she let her gaze move over the children and the earthen patio. Perhaps she was attempting to build rapport with me, an outsider, by distancing herself from the poverty apparent in household we were visiting. However, her clear disdain communicated the stigma of poverty and of being "dirty."

Rural communities face an incredible burden of diarrheal pathogens in the home environment because of a lack of sanitation facilities for the safe disposal of human waste, compounded by a lack of access to clean water within the household. Pit latrines are the most common type of toilet facility available in rural and peri-urban areas of Guatemala. The few new concrete-block homes in Panaj, built with remittances from family working in the United States, have toilets that flush down a pipe and into a pit. In rural areas, there are no sewerage systems, and septic tanks are uncommon. Economic disadvantage and distances from metropolitan centers that have such amenities are to blame—not the hardworking rural population who are shunned for being "dirty" and targeted for endless piecemeal water, sanitation, and hygiene interventions. Just as there have been many types of programs to teach water purification and ORT, there have been projects by bilateral government organizations and NGOs to "improve" latrines. As with most global health programs, some latrines remain in use (see figure 1.2) while others are abandoned in the countryside, either filled in or capped off because they did not support the daily patterns and goals of the family to whom they were given.

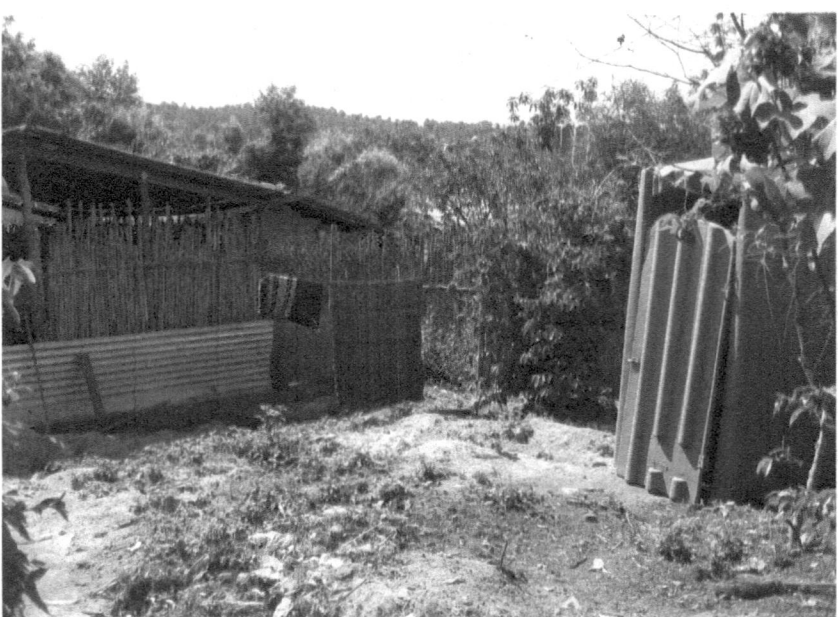

Figure 1.2
A typical pit latrine with an enclosure donated by USAID.

The environment of many communities, particularly rural villages like Panaj, can make identifying diarrhea challenging. Because of the use of latrines, it is difficult to tell when a child has diarrhea after they are potty-trained, since the stool output is typically not visible to caregivers. Most mothers simply describe diarrhea as liquid feces in their children and did not use a specific number of bowel movements per day to define it. The World Health Organization defines diarrhea as three or more loose or watery stools in twenty-four hours, but in a real-world context, it can be impossible—and meaningless—to try to keep track. Mothers in rural Guatemala say diarrhea becomes apparent in children by noticing other symptoms, such as fever, irritability, not wanting to play, and not wanting to eat.

A majority of mothers I spoke with, both Indigenous and ladino, couched their ideas of diarrhea in terms of "dirtiness." Most prominent among all other explanations, I was told that diarrhea is a dirty illness caused by dirty things. Women in even the most rural villages spoke of diarrhea in terms of hygiene and occasionally used germ theory terminology. For example, one mother in a village near Comalapa stated, "I think that if kids get diarrhea it is because of lack of hygiene and cleanliness. Also because flies bring microbes." The speaker here has only three years of schooling and heard about microbes from the health center and understands that they are a "type of dirt that gets spread around." One mother from a village outside of Acatenango explained, "For example, today my daughter told me, 'Mom, look at the water; it's dirty.' From things like this people get diarrhea, and so I would boil water when it looks this way." Most women base their notions of clean and dirty on visible "matter out of place," as Mary Douglas framed it.[83]

The prominent notions of "dirtiness" and lack of hygiene as the causes of diarrhea were consistently accompanied by ideas of the failed or complacent mother. One Maya mother in rural Acatenango aptly described this connection:

> The fact is that some mothers don't clean their children. They don't wash their hands before they eat. They let them play with dirty things that are on the floor. It is then when they get the bacteria and get sick. We blame what they eat. But sometimes children buy food on the street, therefore, we have to know what our children eat, so they don't get germs and end up with diarrhea. We cannot let children play with dirty things. We have to keep them in a clean place. There are careless mothers for whom it is normal that their children play with dirty things. That is how they get sick.

From this explanation of diarrhea, the environment provides sources of possible contamination with a diarrheal illness, but it is ultimately the mother who is to blame. Another woman was even more direct: "Children get diarrhea because mothers are careless." Mothers complain that they cannot watch their children all the time, particularly citing playing and eating outside the household as major sources of diarrheal illness. This functions as a sort of blame-shifting strategy; a mother can still be a "good" mother and have a child with diarrhea if it came from a source outside her control. Women sometimes said that diarrhea was not a problem in their own community but that it was in a neighboring community. These strategies in talking about diarrhea and distancing oneself from it indicate the stigma it carries and its association with poor maternal care.

For all of the pressure put on mothers to have healthy children and enact the standards of "hygiene" from global health water, sanitation, and hygiene programs, the tyranny of "dirtiness" is compounded by racism. The rural Indigenous poor are systematically excluded from social goods and economic advancement in Guatemalan society due to racism. Yet they are tarred and feathered as "backward" and "dirty" for the way of life their position in the social structure affords them, as we saw in the case of mobile nurse looking down at an Indigenous family home. The possible enculturated self-loathing of that nurse, who herself was from a Kaqchikel Maya background, showcases another level of racism and how it is perpetuated. Maya women are subjected to endless lessons on hygiene practices, which often involve instructions and visual depictions that have nothing to do with their lived environments in highland Guatemalan communities; they sit politely while they look at pictures of white hands washing at shiny taps that bear no resemblance to their own water basins. I often think of the soap ads from colonial Britain that read, "The White Man's Burden is through teaching the virtues of cleanliness."[84] This moralizing philosophy and the pervasive notions that only knowledge is lacking and that it is up to an outsider to impart that knowledge remain at the heart of many well-intended but ill-conceived programs to combat diarrhea.

Conclusion

The loss of baby Efraín and the sicknesses threatening Rosario's other children are just a few of the many faces of social suffering within poor Maya communities. Their particular experiences of poor nutritional status and lack of timely access to health care were their own, but their suffering is shared by other children across Guatemala's mountains and the families who try to provide them with care. Just as Maya populations should not be blamed for their own social and economic marginalization, their culture should not be blamed for the failures of biomedicine to serve their communities in general or of ORT programs in particular.

As this chapter has shown, the persistence of the humoral system cannot explain the failures of ORT campaigns in Guatemala. Maya mothers in rural communities with few economic resources are embedded in a health care system where they recognize that better treatments and services are available but not within their reach. They do not have a choice in the kinds of ORT and water, sanitation, and hygiene interventions that target them with instructions, duties, and prohibitions. Moreover, increased exposure to ORT and diarrhea prevention training has introduced concepts of disease transmission and terminology often not fully understood. However, the general concept of hygiene is one of the most primary explanations of diarrhea, leading to the assignment of blame to mothers and their hygiene practices for cases of childhood diarrhea. Chapter 2 further explores women's agency and the intersectionality of gender roles and ethnicity in Guatemala.

2   Entanglements of Empowerment: Women, Caregiving, and Global Health

Oral rehydration therapy is good for preventing blame from not [doing any-thing]. It's always better to have done something than nothing, if you can.
—Kaqchikel Maya mother in Comalapa

We were laughing as I inched my tiny red rental car around the tight moun-tain pass. Rosi joked about how nervous I was driving on the steep dirt road. She stopped fiddling with the radio knob, trying to pick up the stat-icky signal of a romantic ballad coming in from Chimaltenango, to point over the edge of the mountain. "Pull down here," she said. I laughed and said, "No way," glancing at my sleeping infant buckled in the backseat. She smiled and said, "Don't worry. There's really a road; you just can't see the entrance." So I eased over the edge of the cliff, and the car seemed to teeter for a moment before it found the hidden fork in the road to a remote neigh-borhood of her village. "See, you can trust me," she quipped. "I'm a health promoter. *Ixoqí Akunanël* [healing women in Kaqchikel Maya] together!"

I met Rosi when she joined a community-based project to create a group of women health promoters in her village to share information about diar-rhea and oral rehydration therapy (ORT), emphasizing home fluids, with mothers in the community. The promoters were selected by the local village council and helped create the materials they used to teach their peers.[1] That afternoon, we wound our way as far as the rutted dirt road would allow and then walked to get to the home of a community member who was hosting a workshop. Everyone chatted and fussed over my baby, showing him to the nine-month-old little girl of the house as her groom, and eventually all set-tled down for the workshop. I watched Rosi become a woman transformed. At nineteen, Rosi was the youngest member of *Ixoqí Akunanël*, the name the women in this health promoter group chose for themselves, and she was one of the most determined. She took her role as a promoter seriously, and she became animated as she walked the women through the information about ORT and diarrhea. A natural teacher, she knew just when to make a joke and when to ask a question to make sure everyone understood. At the end of the session, everyone thanked Rosi before hurrying home to cook dinner.

Rosi bounced back to the car, excitedly recounting the session and making plans for future ones. I thanked her for all the hard work she was doing. She said, "Of course! I love having something to do—I guess I'm empowered now!" I laughed in the spirit of the moment, but I have thought about this conversation ever since. Rosi was a smart young woman who was at loose ends, reminding me a little of Mercedes, my friend from Panaj who became a nun. She was not married and was trying to save up to go to college to become a teacher. In the meantime, she lived in her parents' household and tended their shopfront, selling chips and soap and other little items to neighbors. I asked her what empowerment meant for her, and she said, "I get to do things! I like to be out in the community, talking to people and doing things. Thank you for making this possible."

It was the thank you that bothered me. Our project had a small amount of grant funding that would run out after a two-year study period. In fact, I felt terrible that we could only give small financial incentives of phone credit to the women in the health promoter group. I did not want be the one—or for her dad to be the one—to give Rosi permission to do the things she wanted. I wanted her to feel empowered all on her own, but I understood that the project gave her a legitimate reason to escape duties at home and do something else for awhile. Rosi did not have many choices, despite her newfound sense of empowerment.

In examining engagement with global health programs more broadly and the use of oral rehydration therapy in particular, the position of women in society and their roles in the family are critical to understanding the hidden impacts of global health. The underbelly of global health includes the uneasy, and too often unexamined, way in which programs can both challenge and reinforce gender inequalities. Within the Guatemalan context, gender-based violence, both through physical and structural violence, constrains Guatemalan women's access to social goods, such as education, judicial processes, and health care. Women's position in society and their ability to effectively navigate the health care system then directly shapes the health care that their children receive. Despite their systemic disadvantages, Maya women draw from their own experiences and the social capital built within their community—the knowledge and support of their peers, elders, and traditional healing systems—to make choices about caring for and treating illnesses in their children.

In this chapter, I explore the patriarchal structures of Guatemalan society and families, which put women on the receiving end of violence, contribute to women's precarity, and perpetuate the expectation that women will do unpaid labor. In doing so, I examine the intersectionality of race and gender in the experiences of Indigenous women. I discuss women's roles as economic contributors within the family, how they manage when men must leave their communities for work, and the unpaid labor of childrearing and navigating care for their families. I further explore how women exert agency, despite these constraints. I conclude with a consideration of the opportunities and burdens that global health programming places on women. At the local level, I consider women's agency in choosing to participate in global health and development programs, and at the global level, I consider gendered patterns of inclusion and marginalization in the design of global health programs within the neoliberal landscape.

Patriarchy and "Women's Place"

Women in Guatemala are largely defined and positioned within the social hierarchy through their relationships with their fathers and husbands. If her father is still living, a woman will be introduced and identified as her father's daughter. I found this to be true of both *ladino* and Indigenous women. Women only become known without reference to male relatives in the community when they are older and recognized for some particular talent or characteristic, such as being an effective healer or midwife. Even then, older women without living husbands may be referred to as the mothers of their sons in local conversations among men or in mixed company when she is not present. Women, of course, refer to their close friends by first names.

Within both ladino and Indigenous households, the senior male is the head of the household. While varying degrees of hierarchical relationships exist between the head of the household, his spouse, and their children, the patriarch is responsible for making major decisions about the family's work, finances, and lifestyle. Indigenous families often live in extended kin groups, with each nuclear family typically having its own room in the household. In this case, a man would make decisions for his immediate family but may have to defer to his father or brothers on matters affecting the entire household.

Women's work and men's work are more clearly divided among ladinos than among the Maya of Chimaltenango.[2] Although fewer Indigenous women say they work outside the home, they may spend much of their time working alongside their husbands in the family's fields. In this respect, they directly contribute to sustaining their families in a way that ladino women often do not. However, both ladino and Indigenous women are solely responsible for the maintenance of the household through cooking, cleaning, and laundering clothes. In fifteen years of fieldwork, I have never seen a husband wash a dish or sweep a floor. Domestic chores are firmly women's work.

Indigenous Women and (Re)production of Maya Culture

The social position of Indigenous women is further complicated in ways that, as this book will demonstrate, affect their access to and uptake of global health interventions. On the national scale, the idea of a woman (much less an Indigenous woman) being a visible political leader threatens the national power structure and *machismo*. When Maya woman and Nobel Peace Prize winner Rigoberta Menchú became visible in the national political arena in the early 2000s, a new genre of joke was born in Guatemala's newspapers that explicitly discusses the probability of Menchú having *huevos* (testicles) under her skirt.[3] The idea that a woman should be involved in public affairs is outside the norm, and the concept of an Indigenous woman doing so is practically unthinkable. Huevos jokes are just one of the leveling mechanisms used to keep Indigenous women in their place. They bear an intersectional double-discrimination that places them at the bottom of Guatemala's social ladder.[4]

In Guatemala, Indigenous clothing (*traje*) and language are the most important markers of ethnic identity. Maya women keep these traditions alive in their families as they care for and enculturate children; even in the face of social exclusion and in contexts of forced migration, they are agentive markers of identity and belonging.[5] While Maya men cannot be identified as Indigenous or ladino by the jeans and cotton shirts that most now wear, Maya women in their brightly colored, intricately woven *huipil* (blouses) and skirts are immediately identified. Diane Nelson described how traje serves as an ethnic and community identity marker:

> *Traje* is supposed to mark specific power differentials in Guatemala. It marks gender (woman versus man), ethnicity (Maya versus ladino), nation (Guatemalan versus foreigner) and class (bourgeois versus worker), as well as internal differences among Mayan peoples, rural people as opposed to urban, and authentic archaic culture as opposed to cosmopolitan modernity.[6]

Maya women are charged with maintenance of Maya culture, and their clothing is the most visible manifestation of this task.

As Cecilia Menjivar has compellingly shown, urban ladina women's lives are patterned by gender-based violence, but it is Maya women who bear the terrible double burden of racism and misogyny that permeates Guatemalan public and private life.[7] Indigenous women's social and physical mobility is curtailed as they are treated as objects of scrutiny and scorn. My friend Juana from Panaj—Flavia's eldest granddaughter—has achieved the dreams that remain unrealized for so many young Maya women. She completed a university degree, continues to work in Guatemala City after her marriage, and shares a home in an urban area with her husband. However, success does not bring safety, and even commuting to and from work in the capital is an ordeal. Juana once told me how she purposely wears the patterned *huipil* of other Maya communities to her workplace so that men there will not know where she is from. The proud marker of her own region becomes a liability.

Maya women also bear the primary responsibility for rearing children to be ethnically Maya by teaching Maya traditions and lifeways. Indigenous women are the makers of corn tortillas, the basis of the Maya diet and central to Maya identity. To eat is to consume tortillas, and any other food is secondary.[8] In the villages, mealtimes are marked by the rhythmic slap-slap-slapping of corn dough into tortillas, which are then toasted on a flat sheet of metal over the fire. In town in Chimaltenango, the houses of Indigenous families are easily discernible by this familiar sound. Maya women model what it is to be Maya to their children through their performance of household chores, their interactions with their spouses, and further, their interactions with the non-Indigenous populations around them. The maintenance of contemporary Maya culture shapes Indigenous women's engagement with public institutions and their health-seeking in ways that are as complicated as the patterns they weave into their textiles.

Violence against Women

It seems so simple to encourage women to attend global health workshops or to take their children to the nearest health facility when they are sick. But these naive directives ignore the fact that every small decision, every journey can be fraught with danger for women. In Guatemala, the quotidian act of leaving home exposes women to violence, and, too often, being inside the home does the same. The gang rape, torture, and mutilation used against Maya women as government counterinsurgency tactics during the internal armed conflict set a hellish precedent for current levels of violent crimes targeting women.[9] The combination of a machismo society that devalues women and a crippled justice system has proved to be deadly. Violent crimes, even homicides, are poorly recorded in Guatemala, and statistics of homicides separated by sex have only been kept since 2001. The 2008 Law against Femicide and Other Forms of Violence against Women further distinguished the crime of femicide, the killing of a woman on the basis of gender. In 2020, eight in 1,000 women and girls experienced violence.[10]

While homicide rates overall have dropped in the last decade, the rate among women has declined less than for men. In 2020, the violent death rate for women was 4.2 in 100,000; an estimated 63.1 in 100,000 women were raped.[11] The bodies of missing women are found mutilated and with obvious signs of sexual violence, and victims are frequently girls under eighteen years of age.[12] Families of victims report that any attempts to pressure the police for an investigation result in recriminations against the victim. When they file a police report, anxious families are often told that their missing relative must have run off with a boyfriend, and investigations center on finding perceived improprieties in the missing person's private life. If and when a body is recovered, authorities and reports in the news media frequently suggest that the woman was a gang member, and her death was the (deserved) result of her gang participation.[13] In response to the growing trend of violence against women, several women's and victim's rights groups have attempted to raise awareness and conduct independent investigations of some cases. Yet, in doing so, they contend with serious resistance: for example, in one week in 2005, twelve investigative offices were ransacked and evidence destroyed.[14] Members of the police have been implicated in some of the crimes against women, which obviously curtails adequate reporting and investigation. It also means that men in positions of authority—police, military, and health providers—may not be trusted.

During the internal armed conflict precipitated by the US-backed military coup of 1954 and only concluded officially in 1996, the rape and torture of Indigenous women was widely used as a weapon of terror and subjugation. Indigenous women were targeted as both supposed helpmeets and members of guerilla forces as well as those capable of producing future Indigenous resistors.[15] Fear kept Indigenous women silent, with few sharing their experiences of rape and brutality at the hands of the Guatemalan army and state-sponsored paramilitary groups beyond close kinship circles.[16] Only now are some Indigenous women seeing possibilities of justice, with a few high-profile cases of war crimes and rape finally coming to trial. The wartime violence perpetrated on women's bodies has had lasting effects on the acceptance of femicide and gender-based violence in contemporary Guatemala.[17]

Of the violence against women, one Guatemalan women's rights activist explains, "Firstly, there is no respect for the body of a woman. People feel they can treat women however they want. Also, there is the idea that women are the property of someone."[18] Crime against women is not taken seriously. Other than homicide rates, no official statistics are kept of gender-based violence. Amnesty International nonetheless reports that sexual and physical abuse in the family, rape, kidnapping, and workplace sexual harassment are serious problems. In fact, the Inter-American Commission on Human Rights has cited Guatemala multiple times for failure to prosecute rape, which is recognized by international law to be a form of torture.[19] Forced marriage and child marriage remain significant issues in Guatemala; nearly 30 percent of women aged 20–24 were married or in a union before age 18.[20]

These alarming rates of violent crime against women keep Guatemalan women from moving freely through public spaces and further confines them to the domestic sphere. Such crimes illustrate to women that they have no recourse should they be victims of violence, particularly if it occurs within their own household. It also justifies male family members' prohibitions against women leaving the household and participating in public life. When women bear the label of "victim" on such a widespread scale, it further reinforces patriarchal norms and prevents women as a group from raising their status in Guatemalan society.[21] None of the women I know would consider traveling even a short distance by bus alone, and women, even in groups, did not leave home after dark.

Incidents of mob violence and vigilante justice reflect the Guatemalan government's weak judicial system, which leads to virtual impunity for criminals. Of 5,338 murders registered by police in 2005, only eight were tried by the criminal justice system.[22] I witnessed the police response immediately after the murder of a well-known neighborhood shopkeeper in an urban area. After they threw the plastic-wrapped body into the back of a truck, they partially rinsed the blood from the street with a couple of buckets of water. It seemed very much business as usual. No formal investigation into the murder was initiated by the police, though rumors quickly circulated that the murder was motivated by robbery and committed by someone outside the neighborhood, which is a mechanism for social distancing from the tragedy. Impunity for gender-based violence remains high. In 2012, only 6.4 percent of complaints of gender-based violence resulted in formal accusations, and only 21 percent of those received a judicial ruling. While criminal impunity has slowly decreased in Guatemala, it remains at an estimated 98 percent for femicide.[23]

High rates of violent crime reinforce suspicion of community outsiders and lack of confidence in governance mechanisms. Families feel that they must protect themselves, and vigilante justice acts as the de facto rule of law. I frequently see men carrying guns in their belt-loops or across their backs, along with the ever-present machetes, which serve as both tool and weapon. In all of the Guatemalan households in which I have spent significant periods of time, furniture or logs were used each night to barricade the street door of the house against forced entry. The opportunities for women and girls to continue education, improve their socioeconomic position, and participate in civic life are severely limited when their ability to leave the home is curtailed by household obligations and fear of personal harm.

Women's Economic Contributions

We have seen that patriarchal familial and social structures reinforce devaluation of women, putting them at risk of violence. The high rates of violence then reinforce those patriarchal norms and limit women's participation in life outside the home. That limitation then makes getting an education and well-paid work incredibly difficult for women, which further puts them under the control of men in their families. The cascade of social forces and structures that ensnare women is complex; yet, women also find avenues for agency, self-determination, and social participation. The limitations and opportunities available to women shape the ways in which they seek health care and engage in global health programs. Here, I consider women's economic position and decision-making roles within household economies. Perhaps most significantly, women spend an average of 20 percent of their time on unpaid domestic labor, limiting their availability for paid work.[24]

I lived for long periods with four families in the Chimaltenango Department whose socioeconomic status ranged from middle class to below the poverty line. It was interesting to observe how household finances were handled. In all cases, each adult had money they considered their own. Rather than putting all money into a communal household fund, husbands and wives discussed who would pay for particular expenses. Apart from the Panaj household, the husbands' earnings were the main sources of income for the households. I did find, however, some differences between ladino and Indigenous households in how women's money was spent.

The ladino households in Chimaltenango and Acatenango were, respectively, lower middle class and more comfortably middle class. In both cases, the wives earned money by doing odd jobs as they came along. In Chimaltenango, Jeny earned money by hosting the occasional gringo volunteer from a local clinic, where she had worked prior to her marriage, and by taking in an occasional typing or data-entry job. Chely in Acatenango took advantage of the lack of restaurants and cafés in town and catered banquet-style meals for friends hosting out-of-town guests. Both women earned their money by working in their own homes at tasks they seemed to enjoy. They spent this money on extras, like new earrings or a treat for their kids. Jeny's husband and father shared the costs of utility bills, and each gave her weekly funds to purchase food at the market. Jeny would often discuss plans to save up and buy things for her young daughter, like a tricycle, and often said was glad that her husband had to pay for things like diapers.

The two Maya families with whom I lived were less well-off than the ladino families. The Comalapa family was working class, while the Panaj family struggled below the poverty line. In Comalapa, three grown children lived in their parents' household in single rooms with their own families.

Doña Nathaly and her daughter-in-law Claudia sewed woven fabric into final products for a weaving cooperative. They used the money they earned to buy things for the household and their children. Although their husbands were the primary providers for the household, their money was still important in keeping the household running. Doña Nathaly kept her earnings separate from her husband's, saying things like, "I'm going to buy a new blanket," and "Don Matteo is going to buy us three bags of maize." In Panaj, money was very scarce, and everyone had to contribute what they could to the household. I once asked a fourteen-year-old cousin of the Panaj family what she planned to do with the money she would earn with her weavings, expecting her to say that she wanted some item for herself from the market in Comalapa. She looked surprised and told me that she would buy maize with her money.

Men (away) at Work

Maya communities no longer have enough land for most families to grow enough food to live a traditional subsistence lifestyle; land rights, of course, were at the heart of the internal armed conflict. Male absenteeism from the home, prompted by compulsory participation in the cash economy for survival, is another key factor shaping women's mobility and choices for health-seeking. Among Maya families living in the rural areas of the Chimaltenango Department, men in the family commonly leave home in search of wage labor in Guatemala City, on plantations on the coasts, or as migrants in the United States. Remittances from relatives working abroad are estimated to be Guatemala's largest foreign currency earner.[25] Though women may sometimes find wage labor in agricultural packing plants and factories, men more often take jobs that keep them away from home.

In Panaj, Estrella and her three small children struggled, alongside her mother-in-law Flavia and sister-in-law Maria, to survive while her husband José was away working in El Norte. José had been away from the village for nearly two years working in the United States on construction sites when I first lived with the family. His transfers of money home had been infrequent, and the women were left to support the family on their own. Flavia and Maria grew maize and beans on the family's plot, which, once dried on the tin roof, provided the basis of the family's diet. Maria's three teenage daughters, Mercedes, Silvia, and Juana, did many of the household chores of sweeping and laundry, and they also spent much of their time weaving to generate income. Estrella cooked and looked after her three small children.

Although they struggled to get by and provide enough food for the children, the women seemed proud to be living on their own. When I first moved in, they proudly welcomed me to their "household of women." Flavia acted as the head of the household, with the others deferring to her opinions about everything from when to plant to how to fix a loom. She was also in charge of selling everyone's weavings at the cooperative's offices in Chimaltenango. Flavia had assumed the role of matriarch and served as the head of the extended family.

Finally, José returned from the United States. Chickens were killed, and male village elders were invited to the house for a celebratory lunch. It was a joyous occasion as José met his almost two-year-old son for the first time, with woodsmoke and the celebratory sounds of marimba on the radio wafting above the patio. The household, particularly José's own nuclear family, was going to be much better off now that he had returned with money earned in the United States and could work in the family's fields. Soon after his return, I noticed that José was acting as head of the household and that Flavia was asking him about things, like when to go into town to the market, which the others had recently been asking her. Though José was good-natured and respectful of his mother, wife, and sister, it was clear that they were no longer a household of women and that the patriarch had returned. This illustrates a pattern found in many Guatemalan households: women make day-to-day decisions about household finances and childcare, but when it involves a larger expenditure or a possible trip to town, the men are typically consulted.

Education and Opportunities for Women

Limitations on women's education hinder not only economic opportunities but also make health care decision-making and engagement with global health programs more challenging. While women's literacy rates in Guatemala have reached parity with men's at about 80 percent, girls are far less likely to complete secondary education or university, which often involves travel outside of small communities to urban areas. The relatively high national literacy rates obscure rural/urban and Indigenous/ladino disparities.[26] For many rural Maya women, lack of schooling outside their community also means that they are unable to communicate easily in Spanish, limiting their abilities to easily participate in the marketplace economy.

One important way that Maya women have overcome these barriers to work is through participation in weaving cooperatives. Through weaving cooperatives, started as development projects by foreign nongovernmental organizations (NGOs), women sell their weavings at a fair price. Their woven cloth is then finished into a final product and sold in tourist markets or exported.[27] Through weaving cooperatives, women get to earn money by using a skill that they already have and that they can do while still fulfilling their household obligations and caring for their children (see figure 2.1).

Weaving is a strong identity marker and a source of pride for Indigenous women. Each region in Guatemala has a distinctive style of huipil, and women will often work with their mothers and sisters on a single intricate huipil for up to two years. To be able to have a small collection of huipiles serves not only as an identity marker as Maya but also as a status symbol. Even more importantly, weaving is women's work and is highly

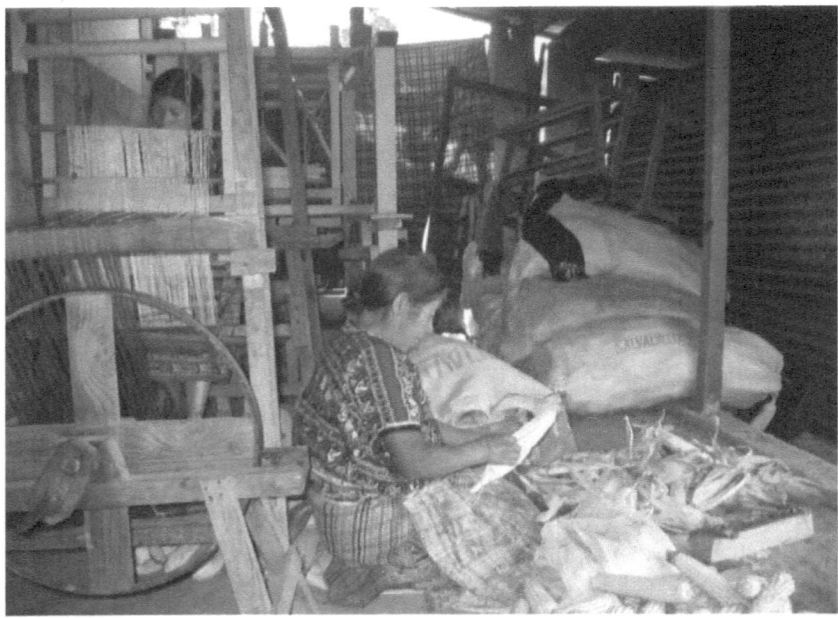

Figure 2.1
Women's work in Panaj.

valued for both the skill required and the money that it can earn. In the Maya households where I lived in Comalapa and Panaj, women's hands were always busy with weaving or spinning thread. I began to crochet hats and scarves to have something to keep my own hands busy while I sat and talked with women. Many afternoons, after putting aside piles of files and notes from my research, I would go outside to enjoy a welcome break from my work to crochet and chat. Several times, I was greeted with, "Oh, you're (finally) going to do your work now." The generative process of weaving is women's work, not shuffling through paperwork.

Women, particularly rural Maya women, must look hard for economic opportunities to help support themselves and their families. While there is a growing middle class of Maya and ladino women achieving higher education and entering the formal workforce, household occupations continue to be an important source of income for rural Maya women. Weaving is a key economic activity accessible to them, though it would be impossible to support a family with earnings from weaving alone. Indigenous women also sell tortillas to other better-off households, for whom buying tortillas and skipping the labor-intensive processes of grinding the corn, making the dough, and patting out endless circles over the fire is a desirable convenience. Women also sometimes take in laundry for money. For women in Panaj, like Rosario who lost her baby and has an abusive, unreliable husband, supporting a family is a challenge that requires ceaseless labor, both paid and unpaid.

Women's Unpaid Labor

The afternoon found us once again on the earthen patio of Doña Flavia's home. The radio played a lively mix of merengue and romantic ballads, to which Estrella's lively six-year-old son would dance with hilarious exaggeration and flair. A tiny village Casanova! His little four-year-old sister and toddler brother laughed along and wandered about the courtyard finding all sorts of amusements, from splashing in the water basin to taunting the chickens in their coop. The constant, ceaseless backdrop to the children's play, forming a rhythmic counterpart to the music, was their mother Estrella's *scrub-scrub-scrubbing* of the family's laundry against the ridged surface of the concrete washbasin. She scrubbed, rinsed, and twisted diapers, tiny clothes, woven skirts and blouses, and heavy blankets and then hung them to dry in the sun. It took hours.

Like other communities across the Guatemalan highlands, the cash-poor households of Panaj were often at the cusp of utter destitution, particularly in the late summer season when harvest was still a few months away. The typical daily diet consists of corn tortillas and weak coffee for breakfast and dinner and a lunch of tortillas, beans, eggs, and the occasional pot of boiled foraged herbs. Most families keep chickens, though they are slaughtered only on special occasions, and the few families who keep pigs sell them for cash in Comalapa rather than consume them. While Estrella's husband was away working in the United States, the family was living in a state of constant food insecurity, though the women continued to grow corn and sell weavings. Estrella's three children were small for their ages and constantly irritable with hunger, frequently crying themselves to sleep at night and begging their mother for more food that simply was not available—not in their home, not in their village.

Estrella's struggle to make ends meet and care for her children is the daily struggle played out across Guatemala. Women are the primary caregivers of children and bear the responsibility of feeding them. Yet the limited choices available to rural Maya women for education and earning make this a daunting prospect in many households. Global health programs often aim to provide resources and opportunities for exactly these groups of women, but these programs often fail to consider the structural realities into which they are so hopefully inserted. Cheerful posters on how to wash hands make no sense when the sink basin and soap depicted in training materials are curiosities absent from women's lives. Such offerings become laughable when so much time must be dedicated just to getting enough to eat.

Of particular importance for global health nutrition and oral rehydration therapy campaigns is an understanding of child feeding practices and the unpaid labor that women do to feed their children. Most Guatemalan mothers I talked to, both ladino and Indigenous, said they breastfed their babies exclusively for between six to nine months. Ladino mothers introduce grains and grain beverages (*atol*), followed by vegetables and other foods that the rest of the family is eating. In comparison, mothers in Panaj introduce foods other than breastmilk to their children when they reached six to thirteen months, and they continue to give breastmilk in addition to other foods until the child is up to two years old. In the village setting, children are almost exclusively kept wrapped and in a sling with their mothers or another female relative until their first birthday, facilitating on-demand feeding. While packaged atol beverages were popular among ladino mothers for young children up to five years of age, I never saw a Maya mother give one of these beverages to her child. [28] This is in spite of the fact that free bags of powdered atol were given out to pregnant women and children under three years of age in rural villages as part of a nutrition supplementation project of the UN World Food Programme. The time when a child is being weaned and learning to walk, between the ages of one and two years, is particularly fraught with the peril of diarrhea, and most of the rural mothers I spoke with felt diarrhea was an inevitable part of this stage of development. They did, however, feel that certain foods were helpful in seeing the child safely through this period.

Mothers in Panaj most frequently cited rice, beans, pasta, and eggs as good foods for a child being weaned. They said there was no difference in foods that were good for girls and boys, and they wean both at the same age. However, for slightly older children, equality in the amount and type of food seems to change. For example, on a couple of occasions, the six-year-old boy in my household in Panaj stole his little sister's food when their mother was not looking. When his sister started crying, punishment was swift for the both of them—her for complaining, him for stealing—and the assumption was that the little boy needed the food more. In this very resource-poor environment, mothers were not able to consistently give their children the diet they felt was most healthy for them. Several mothers I talked to said that it was good to give children meat (chicken or sausages) once or twice a week, but I observed that families in the village did not consume meat more than once or twice a month. However, children were given preferential access to eggs, eating them once or twice a day. Eggs are held to be very nutritious for children and to help build strength. In addition to eggs, village children primarily ate corn tortillas and beans.

The Burdens of "Dirtiness" and Diarrhea

Mothers often recognized that hygiene practices, like handwashing and keeping a clean latrine, would help protect their children from diarrhea. However, the pace of life and living conditions make these measures difficult to implement in reality. In Flavia, Estrella, and Maria's joint household in Panaj, children's hands were rarely washed because the patio where they play is packed dirt, so it feels futile. The women said that they did not clean the latrine because "it just goes down into the ground anyway," but every couple of days they carefully burned the newsprint and corncobs used in place of toilet paper. Housekeeping duties are taken very seriously, including sweeping the dirt floors and patio clean of debris every day and hand-laundering clothes, but children are bound to get dirty, so it was a pointless effort to try to always keep them clean.

It is only when a child falls ill that a mother's hygiene and care of her child comes under scrutiny. Obviously, no mother wants to be known as someone who keeps a dirty household and whose children persistently get diarrhea. One mother in Panaj summed up the social pressure women are under to keep a clean home and healthy children, saying, "Children get diarrhea because mothers are careless. They don't give them healthy food, and things are left dirty. This is what causes diarrhea." These self-blaming attitudes are the ghosts of global health programs past, which intended to train women in water, sanitation, and hygiene but failed to create the infrastructure and environment where their instructions could actually be implemented. The resulting stigma and social pressures serve to delay treatment-seeking outside the home in an effort to conceal cases of diarrhea.

During focus group discussions and in-depth individual interviews, I asked mothers at what time of the year and during which stages of child development diarrhea is the greatest problem. Nearly everyone mentioned the beginning of the "winter" or the start of the rainy season in May. Most explanations for this timing centered on the concept that there is "too much air" at the start of the rainy season and that the rains churn up all the dust, mixing germs into the water. One mother observed, "Yes, every year in the month of May is when many children die because of diarrhea. This is because it starts raining, and the worms in children get disturbed and the diarrhea begins." Though a less prominent response, a few women also noted the "rotavirus season" in November to January.

Guatemalan mothers frequently say that diarrhea begins somewhere between eight months and one year, when children begin to crawl and start putting dirty things in their mouths. About half of mothers I interviewed also said that diarrhea is common between twelve and fourteen months, when children are teething. Also, between one and two years of age, children are weaned off breastmilk, and mothers noted that diarrhea frequently accompanies this process. Both in terms of seasonality and developmental stages, the responses of mothers in my sample reflect previous research on the classification of diarrhea in rural Guatemala.[29] Of particular importance, Elizabeth Burleigh and colleagues noted that when diarrhea is associated with a developmental milestone, it may be classified as a symptom of growth rather than a sickness in its own right; therefore, such cases of diarrhea may not be treated.[30] Childhood diseases and the undernutrition that underpins poorer outcomes from disease have been normalized within rural Maya communities because of entrenched structural violence and systems of exclusion.[31] Maya communities have been forced to accept that their children will be sick, but they agentively choose treatments across the traditional, private, and public health sectors.

Navigating Decisions on Health-Seeking for Children

Claudia was a twenty-three-year-old Maya woman who lived with her husband, two-year-old daughter, and seven-month-old son in Comalapa. They lived in two rooms in the household of her parents-in-law, along with her husband's two brothers, sister, and nephew. They used one room, equipped with a stove, as a kitchen and the second room as a sitting room and bedroom. The family as a whole can best be described as an up-and-coming working-class Maya family. Claudia's in-laws have instilled the value of education in their children, and each has gone on to career-training or university after completing secondary school. Claudia's husband Alvaro was attending a university course in Guatemala City, where he commutes daily from Comalapa. Although Alvaro and his siblings grew up in fairly humble circumstances, the material wealth of the family has increased as they have entered the formal workforce. The house has been expanded to nearly double in size by different siblings to accommodate their own families within the household, and Alvaro's sister paid for the addition of a water storage tank and large pila.

Claudia was a cheerful person, secure in her close relationships with her in-laws, happy in her marriage, and content with her material lifestyle. Although Claudia and Alvaro had less money than Alvaro's other siblings because he is in school, they were able to get by on the money from his part-time job. They both looked forward to a time when Alvaro could spend more time at home and when money would not be so tight, but they planned to continue living in his parents' household in Comalapa. With the greater income that Alvaro will earn, Claudia said they plan to give their own children a good education and, in time, make improvements and additions to the household. Claudia finished secondary school but did not work outside the home. She delighted in her two children, spending the day singing to them and teaching her two-year-old new things as she went about her household chores.

Claudia told me that she does not go to the health center unless she really must. She said that the health center made her feel uncomfortable and that she liked to treat her children's illnesses at home as much as possible. During the national measles vaccine campaign that took place while I was living in Claudia's household, Claudia refused to go get her injection, even though her mother-in-law and sisters-in-law reminded her and gently cajoled her about it several times. She said that she is happiest at home and did not want to go all the way to the health center (a fifteen-minute walk into town) just to get a "sting." Claudia also told me that if one of her children was very sick and needed a doctor, she would more than likely go to a private doctor in Chimaltenango, even if she had to borrow money from one of her in-laws. In fact, both of her sisters-in-law took their children to a private doctor in Chimaltenango. They said the doctor there knew their kids and their family and provided a better quality of care than the health center. In this sense, Claudia may have been discouraged from using the health center, although it is close to her home and free, because it is not considered to be of high quality. Claudia, like most parents, wants to *provide* the best care she can to her children; further, she wants to be *perceived* as providing the best possible care for her children.

Claudia's own upbringing emphasized the use of traditional treatments and belief in the humoral elements of many sicknesses. Claudia did not adhere strictly to the traditional system of carefully selecting foods for their humoral properties, but she believed that hot–cold imbalance can cause fever and diarrhea in children. During my time in her household, Claudia did not visit a traditional healer, although one lives a few houses away, but she did use traditional humoral treatments for her children at home on two different occasions. She said she prefers to use these at-home treatments that her mother used instead of visiting a healer; if the children became more ill, then she would take them to a doctor.

The first occasion Claudia used a traditional remedy was when her two-year-old daughter Nathaly developed a fever and, later, a cough. The fever began the day after the wedding of one of Claudia's cousins, where about 200 friends and relatives had been crowded together in the courtyard of a family member's house for the festivities. Nathaly spent the day running and playing with the other kids at the wedding. When she developed a fever the next day, Claudia explained that it was likely caused by the great heat generated by the crowd of wedding guests; Nathaly had gotten excess heat from them. She put green herbs, *ruda* and *chilka*, that she gathered on the hillside surrounding the house into a knit cap on Nathaly's head. Claudia said that the cool herbs would draw the excess heat and, therefore, the fever out of Nathaly. Two days later, when Nathaly also developed a cough, Claudia put the same herbs in a cloth tied around Nathaly's stomach and chest. The cough was just a further sign that the excess heat had taken hold and needed to be balanced by the cooling effects of the herbs. Nathaly's symptoms persisted for about a week, but the herbs and the watchful eye of Claudia were the only treatments given to her.

Also, during my stay in the household, Nathaly's seven-month-old brother Emilio got diarrhea. Claudia was not overly concerned with the onset of the diarrhea, since she had begun introducing new foods other than breastmilk. She said, "It's to be expected a little bit at his age, poor thing. When you start giving them different food, their little stomachs have to adjust, and sometimes they don't like the food." Even when Emilio's diarrhea persisted for three days, Claudia remained untroubled: he was a strong, healthy baby, and he continued to nurse during the bout of diarrhea. On the fifth day, Claudia started to worry more, since Emilio was becoming more irritable and difficult to feed. She took a raw egg and passed it over Emilio's stomach. The egg was then cracked into a dish to check its color: if it has color, it has been "cooked" by the heat in the child's body, and the heat has effectively been removed. Claudia judged Emilio's egg to have an orange "cooked" color and felt that this had sufficiently cooled him.[32] This was the only treatment given to Emilio during his bout of diarrhea, which lasted a total of seven days.

While Claudia preferred to use home treatments instead of going to the health center or doctor, she recognized the value of biomedicine in treating more serious conditions or sicknesses that do not respond to at-home care. In the case of Emilio's diarrhea, she did not make or purchase an oral rehydration solution, but she did say that it was important to keep children hydrated during diarrhea, hence her efforts to continue to breastfeed Emilio during his sickness. She felt that ORT would be important for a child who was not breastfeeding who had a particularly "strong" case of diarrhea.

While mothers may initially use home remedies, humoral beliefs do not prevent mothers from using biomedical treatments. Nearly all mothers who mentioned humoral conceptions of diarrheal illness did not report delayed biomedical treatment-seeking beyond the normal waiting period of other mothers in their communities. In a survey I conducted at community gatherings in the Chimaltenango Department in 2006 and 2007, I found that most mothers recognized the danger of allowing a severe case of diarrhea to go on for too long a time; of 307 participants, 17 percent termed diarrhea a "dangerous" illness, and 20 percent associated diarrhea with dehydration. In fact, traditional healers often encourage further treatment-seeking and support women in navigating their choices. Traditional healers are an important locus of women's agency and power within communities.

In addition to women who are humoral healers (*curanderas*), lay midwives (*comadronas*) occupy important positions of trust, leadership, and maternal caregiving within Maya communities, where there is a strong cultural preference for giving birth in the home because of tradition and well-founded fears of racist treatment within biomedical facilities.[33] Claudia's navigation between traditional healing and biomedical care in institutional settings that were not comfortable to her reflects the decision-making process many Maya women undertake, though Claudia had greater financial resources and geographic access to care than most.

Realities of Administering ORT

Giving ORT is hard work. Posters and training materials from global health organizations and the Guatemalan Ministry of Health all show women gently holding a cup or spoon to the lips of a willing, relaxed child. But that is not reality. In fact, preventing diarrhea and giving ORT requires additional unpaid household labor from women. Diarrhea prevention training programs ask women to implement water purification, household cleaning, and handwashing strategies they often do not have the time or resources to do. ORT itself requires supplies, time, and persistence. It is not so simple.

After decades of various ORT interventions, most mothers, Maya and ladino, in the Chimaltenango Department have heard about ORT. Yet, hearing about its benefits does not make it easy to give to a child. Ninety-two percent of mothers, when directly asked during individual survey interviews, said that they felt ORT was "good" or "effective" for diarrhea.[34] Even among women who said they believed ORT is good, incorrect ideas about what ORT does and how it works were common. For example, those who believed that ORT stopped diarrhea indicated that they have either never used ORT (and seen the increased stool output that it causes) or never used ORT in sufficient quantity. One mother in Panaj said, "ORT washes the stomach, and it stops the diarrhea." Others believed that ORT replaces nutrition for a child with diarrhea, and therefore they may withhold other foods from the child during diarrhea. There are many possible causes for these misperceptions about ORT and what it is supposed to do. I found that, in attempting to promote ORT, health workers occasionally misinform mothers by telling them that ORT is what they need to "cure" or "fix" a case of diarrhea. Simplifying explanations of ORT to this level may lead to non-use of ORT after an initial trial fails to yield the expected curative results and can even be dangerous in the case of food withholding.

Preparing and Storing Oral Rehydration Solutions

Mothers who said ORT was not good explained that it simply does not work. They said ORT did not make their children get better and that it made the (volume of) diarrhea worse. This again illustrates that misunderstanding the purpose and function of ORT leads mothers to feel that it does not work. Misunderstandings of the function of ORT can also be dangerous among mothers who felt positively toward ORT. In two interviews, mothers indicated that they had used laxative enemas for children with diarrhea. They both cited the commonly held view that ORT was a good way to "clean out" the stomach, evidenced by the increased stool output that ORT causes. This indicates a belief that ORT and laxatives create the same effect and can, therefore, be used interchangeably. This misconception has obvious dire consequences for levels of dehydration and nutritional status in children with diarrhea.

The way to prepare packets of oral rehydration salts (ORS), as recommended by health center doctors and mobile teams in the Chimaltenango Department, is to mix the contents of a packet with one liter of boiled or chlorinated water. Apart from using rinsed-out plastic soda bottles, most mothers in rural areas do not have ways of measuring the correct amount of water. Most women who told me they had used ORS packets said that they tended to estimate the right amount of water by tasting the solution. They might mix up the solution in a cooking pot or prepare an individual serving in a cup by mixing in just a small portion of the packet. If mothers mix the ORS packets with water incorrectly, their children are not getting the benefits of oral rehydration therapy. Given that the health posts tend to give only one or two packets of ORS at a time, mothers most likely use the ORS powder too sparingly, negating the benefits of optimal electrolyte absorption. However, if ORS solution is mixed with too little water, it can exacerbate dehydration due to the salt content.

Although ORT guidelines recommend that ORT be given to children even if the water used to make them is not purified, this can expose children to additional pathogens when their immune systems are already fighting a diarrheal infection. Only about 20 percent of the women I interviewed used bottled, boiled, or chlorinated drinking water in their households, and they would use the same water source to prepare ORT. In the past ten years, piped water has been made available in some of the smaller villages in Chimaltenango, including Panaj. However, the water in Panaj is still untreated, and local men sometimes bathe in the lagoon that is the source of piped water. Because it is untreated and exposed to environmental contaminants, piped water may have the same or even higher levels of diarrheal pathogens than streams or other flowing sources of water. Yet the fact that water comes from a pipe leads rural women to reasonably believe that it is clean and safe for drinking.

Another component of safe administration of ORT is knowing when to discard leftover solution. Out of about seventy mothers participating in focus groups, only two knew that ORS solution should be thrown away twenty-four hours after it has been mixed.[35] Again, paucity of free packets available at health posts and from community health workers would make it counterintuitive for women who are accustomed to wasting nothing to throw away leftover solution. Several times, women have proudly showed me the remains of an ORS bottled solution sitting on a windowsill or shelf in their homes, often with months of dust and grime accumulated on the container.

The time commitment that it takes to administer ORT to children is also often beyond what mothers can provide. Health centers and mobile teams recommend that children be given a half a glass of ORT every hour or two spoonfuls every fifteen minutes for very young children. This is a labor-intensive endeavor, particularly for rural Maya women who are more likely to be performing manual labor in fields away from the household. Also, the large family size in many Maya households makes it difficult to devote the time needed to effectively administer ORT when there are many other children who require care and attention.

Child Resistance to ORT and Force-Feeding

Remember that about 70 percent of the population of the Chimaltenango Department cannot meet their basic nutritional needs. Given these high levels of undernutrition, the effects of repeated bouts of infectious disease, particularly diarrhea, exacerbate poor nutritional status and inhibit childhood growth and development.[36] When children are undernourished, they often become irritable and lethargic. As undernutrition progresses, they become apathetic, refusing food and showing little interest in or response to the world around them.[37] The presence of this level of undernutrition in Chimaltenango became glaringly clear to me one afternoon when I was with the mobile health team in a small plantation village outside of Acatenango. The team was attempting to keep children up to date on their vaccine schedules, and they were knocking on doors to seek out the children on their list. When one visibly nutritionally wasted two-year-old girl got her vaccination while lying in her mother's arms, she did not cry at all; she barely turned her head to look at the injected arm and frowned. The mother said that the girl did not like to play or eat anymore, and the team's nurse told her that she must try to force her to eat or at least drink some atol.

Of course, we know that healthy two-year-olds cry when they get vaccinated. After I noticed the severe apathy and very apparent undernutrition in this little girl, I began to notice other rural children having the same response to their vaccines and the same signs of undernutrition. The childrearing approach common in many rural Maya households prioritizes soothing young children and makes it counterintuitive for mothers to force-feed their children when they fight it, particularly for a foul-tasting ORS solution. Moreover, mothers may not recognize that force-feeding is crucial if a child reaches stages of dehydration and undernutrition to the point of severe apathy, where the child is no longer crying or demanding attention. A mother in Panaj stated, "When kids have diarrhea, they don't eat. It's not good to force them. They get sicker if they eat something they don't want." The sentiment that children who have diarrhea should just be given the food that they want was echoed by one of her neighbors in a separate interview, "When a child has diarrhea, they just eat a little of whatever they like—like vegetables. They almost don't eat tortillas at all."

A few mothers who discussed force-feeding said that they attempted to force-feed by using a plastic syringe they had been given, along with an ORS packet, at the health post. They said use syringes to push the solution into their children's mouths when they are refusing to drink. One woman showed me her syringe, kept on a dusty window ledge along with a half-used bottle of premixed solution, that she had gotten from the health center a couple of years before. The results of a study conducted in Comalapa found that a primary risk factor for diarrhea in children was the use of bottles for feeding since the bottles and their rubber nipples were typically not properly sanitized.[38] It stands to reason that the same problem would hold for syringes used in force-feeding ORT, and the promotion of the use of syringes to administer ORT may have hidden dangers. Clearly, it takes more than a few packets of oral rehydration salts to improve childhood diarrhea outcomes, just as it takes more than a workshop on empowerment to improve women's options.

Selective Care and Family Planning

I would be remiss if I did not briefly discuss family planning and family size in relation to the cascade of patriarchal social structures and marginalization in which Maya women live and raise their children. When faced with incredibly limited resources, mothers must make choices on how those resources will be expended and how food and treatment-seeking will be prioritized for different members of the household. The one example of selective withdrawal of care that I witnessed was Rosario with baby Efraín, described in the book's introduction. She did not actively leave her baby exposed to the elements or withdraw food, but she did seem to understand on the afternoon that I spent with her that he would die if he did not receive further medical attention. Yet, she made the decision—if one can truly call it that, given her lack of options—to seek no further treatment for her baby. She felt she could not in good conscience spend further time or money treating an already gravely sick infant when she had eight other hungry children to feed. Caroline Brettell calls into question Western concepts of "neglect" and "infanticide" and argues that these terms make an absolute value judgment on caregiver's actions, regardless of circumstance and intentionality. Brettell's discussion of the complex balance that women have to maintain between income-generating activities and caregiving in order to ensure the survival and success of her children is particularly applicable to the case of Rosario.[39] Given extremely scant resources, Rosario could not pursue every possible treatment for Efraín at the expense of being able to care for her other children, but she did not want him to die.

In such resource-poor environments as the rural villages of Chimaltenango, choices do have to be made about what kind of care is possible for each child and for the family as a whole. In Panaj, Estrella cannot buy her children the sausages she thinks are good for them each week, but she feeds them eggs and gets sausages when she can. There are constant choices between what is best for now and what would be best for the future, like spending money on much-needed extra food or being able to pay school fees. Most mothers do not make decisions about food allocations within the household autonomously; rather, their husbands and mothers-in-law play a key role in shaping how food is distributed.[40] Food is often shared within households by prioritizing the needs of those who are viewed as contributing most to the labor of the household, typically adult men. Children who have been identified as undernourished by health services are often not given more food than other children in the same age range.[41] Further, boys are frequently perceived as being hungrier and requiring more food than girls, resulting in gendered differences in growth and undernutrition.[42] The embodied outcomes of gender disparities start at birth.

Family size also shapes women's opportunities and their caregiving responsibilities. Family planning is difficult to access and to navigate within relationships. Abortion is illegal in Guatemala, and condoms have been difficult to promote in a machismo culture where men often believe a wife's desire to use condoms indicates she is having an affair. Access to contraception has nearly doubled in the past twenty years to 49 percent among married women.[43] However, like most metrics in Guatemala, this number obscures the disparities in access between rural and urban and Maya and ladino populations. The most common types of birth control used in rural Chimaltenango communities are long-acting hormonal implants and IUDs. These have the advantage of lasting for months to years at a time and being easier to conceal from a partner than contraceptive pills. The Guatemalan government partners with Planned Parenthood Global on family planning programs, and NGOs also provide expanded services. Within the Chimaltenango Department and beyond, the NGO WINGS (Asociación Alas de Guatemala) provides essential access to family planning methods, including long-acting methods of contraceptives and permanent choices of both male and female sterilization.

Still, rural women who are interested in limiting the size of their family have inadequate access to the information and materials they need, controlled by limited government resources and, closer to home, the desires of their partners. "I know some women do things. How do you keep from having children? I have too many children, and I cannot take care of them the way that I would like to," said a mother of eleven in Panaj. In talking with women, I often found them to be curious about how various methods worked, and they typically seemed genuinely interested in how to limit their fertility. During a focus-group discussion in Panaj, the conversation drifted from diarrheal treatments when the women learned that I was married and did not yet have children at the time:[44]

Felicita: Where are your kids? Don't you have any?

Rachel: We don't have any yet, but we want to have kids in a few years.

Clemencia: Maybe she can't have any?

Estrella: What do you do to not have children?

Myrna [research assistant]: Everyone is curious about how you don't have kids.

Rachel: I take a pill every day that keeps me from having children, and I will stop taking it when we do want kids.

Estrella: Oh, we knew a woman, Ester, who took those pills, and she died. They made her have miscarriages all of the time, and then she got a big tumor in her womb and died.

Rachel: I'm not sure what happened to your friend, but the pills are pretty safe, and they don't make me sick. There are other methods to keep from having babies, too, like condoms. Have you heard of those?

Felicita: [*Giggling*] Our husbands won't use those. They'll think we have boyfriends if we want to use those. [*More laughter.*]

Estrella: I tried timing with my period [rhythm method], but it didn't work.

During this discussion and others, women expressed that they had too many kids, which kept them from providing for them the way they wanted. Unfortunately, lack of information, fears of infertility and side effects, and lack of partner and familial support are enduring barriers to increased use of contraceptives in Chimaltenango.[45]

Within the Guatemalan social hierarchies that minimize the presence of Maya populations, Maya adolescent girls and women only become visible within government health programming as mothers and potential mothers.[46] They become valuable to the neoliberal state only as producers of future labor. The sole government health programs for adolescent girls and women of reproductive age are those focused on safe maternity and improving the health of the children they bear. Important critiques have been raised about the popular global health nutrition program focused on the first thousand days of life, covering the period from conception to the child's second birthday, which was adopted as a program by the Guatemalan Ministry of Health in partnership with the World Food Programme and other global partnerships. This program exclusively focuses on the health outcomes of the child rather than also considering adolescent mothers as children themselves, with their own physical and developmental needs.[47] Maternity is reinforced as the only value that Maya women bring to society through this exclusive focus on maternal health and the elision of mothers as people.[48]

My Positionality as a Woman in Guatemala

We have seen that women, particularly Maya women, are devalued in Guatemalan society. I cannot complete this discussion of the position of Guatemalan women, their roles in the family, and their challenges in caregiving and health-seeking without acknowledging and discussing my own status as a gringa working in Guatemala. In my privilege as a white foreigner, I experience my identity as a woman in Guatemala very differently than both my ladino and Maya friends and colleagues. I am often awarded a pragmatic (and problematic) honorary status as a man so that I am able to undertake activities and navigate spaces that most Guatemalan women would not.[49] I have realized that I play the part, typically dressing in loose pants and button-down shirts to avoid attracting attention from men. The masculine-perceived attire adopted by foreign women working in Guatemala often elicits jokes and offers of more attractive clothing (which was my experience in Panaj).[50] Once, I was walking with a male Maya colleague through a more dangerous part of town in Chimaltenango at dusk after we had finished up a day of work. He joked that he felt safe walking with me because of the assertive way I was walking, saying no one would want to mess with me. I hoped so.

I also find myself routinely adopting the safety strategies of local women, such as not going out alone or after dark. I constantly consider how to stay safe in a place where women are not valued and where, by default, I stand out. Fieldwork in anthropology and global health implicitly values risk-taking and bravado in ways that undermine commitments to gender equity and can further complicate and obscure our relationships as fieldworkers to local communities.[51] Women's bodies in the field and in the commission of global health programming become objects of scrutiny and loci for the maintenance of the status quo. In urban Chimaltenango, I have often been catcalled, sometimes followed by men in the street, and once pulled into an alley in an attempted assault.[52] Global health research and implementation programs largely ignore the risks to women fieldworkers, both local and foreign, particularly as they rely on the labor of women to implement programming that often goes against local gender norms.[53]

I always begin work in new communities through a snowballed network of contacts, and I now enjoy the benefits of long-term work in the region, where I am well-known in many communities and among local health and development organizations. Even so, a woman working away from home is a curiosity. I have often explained that I need to be in Guatemala as a part of my work, which seems to resonate in rural communities where Maya men, and increasingly women, temporarily move away from their homes to perform agricultural wage labor on the coasts, construction and other labor jobs in Guatemala City, or migrate to the United States. Over the years, I have found that people are very curious to meet my husband—this man who would let his unaccompanied wife stray so far from home. Later, after I had children of my own who traveled with me for fieldwork, Guatemalan women have supported me with offers to hold and feed my children, give advice, and commiserate on the challenges of mothering. My questions about children, growth, nutrition, and diarrhea no longer seemed so strange! Mothering as a global health fieldworker offers its own host of opportunities and challenges.[54]

It has been the privilege of my lifetime to build deep friendships and working partnerships in Chimaltenango and beyond in Guatemala since I first visited in 2005. I love that so many hearths feel like home. But I recognize that they are not my home, and I struggle with the unearned privileges that have brought me to those seats by the fire and inevitably shaped my worldview. For example, my first experience with food insecurity was when

I lived in Panaj with Flavia, Estrella, Maria, and Mercedes. There were only a couple of small shops in Panaj with a few chips, cookies, and sodas. You could not buy any other food there. Flavia's household was representative of many others that worked hard in their fields every day to grow enough to eat because limited transportation and lack of money meant trips to the market in Comalapa for food were rare. When we discussed me moving into her household, Flavia told me bluntly, "There's no food for you here. You'll have to bring your own." I had the ability to go to the market weekly and the *quetzales* to buy what I wanted, even on a small research budget. I would strategize all week on how much food I could buy at the market and carry back to the village.

In the household, we settled into a pattern of communal cooking and food-sharing. Beyond the logistical challenges of getting food, I wrestled with how to balance being authentically present in Panaj, to understand life in the village, without playacting poverty. So many ethnographers before me have struggled with encountering poverty, not as an exotic other but as the horribly mundane backdrop against which the lives of the global majority are lived.[55] To sit, to see, to start to understand the worlds of others was an incredible gift, but my passport and return airline ticket were always right there, tucked away in my backpack. During my time in Panaj, I became hungry, skinny, and tired, but I chose every moment of it. The women in Flavia's household had no tickets, no backpacks, few quetzales, and fewer choices. I am and will always be an outsider, and I try to navigate this position with respect and gratitude. However, I recognize that my presence during fieldwork and the differences in wealth, power, and privilege between me and my interlocutors are a part of the complex and problematic web of power dynamics in global health.

Women as Targets of Global Health

Guatemalan women are most often positioned as passive recipients by global health and development programs that need and expect them to turn information into action and to make programs successful. They are also recruited as volunteers or low-paid community health workers to do the hard work of community implementation of global health initiatives. The ability to take on these tasks is shaped and constrained by the inequalities women face in Guatemalan society—and doubly so for Indigenous

Maya women. The patterns we have seen in Guatemala women's engagement with the health system and global health programming are repeated around the world. Global health programs have "gendered discourses of deservingness" through which women are framed as instruments—of maternity, of targets of programs, and as unpaid labor.[56] Most global health programs in Guatemala are conceived by foreign donors and planned in Guatemala City by men but delivered in marginalized rural and peri-urban communities by women. This reflects global health structures through which men from high-income countries lead programs and women deliver them.[57]

Maya women are most often the targets of global health programs in poor rural areas. The intersectionality of their identities as both women and Indigenous—living within social structures that are both misogynous and racist—profoundly shapes their experiences of engaging with social goods like health services. Global health programs are necessarily overlaid on top of deep historical roots that have produced current inequities. Contemporary gender-based violence is a continuation of historical patterns begun at conquest and pursued with genocidal zeal throughout the Guatemalan colonial period, including targeted rape of Indigenous women to whiten the population.[58] This is how "development" began in Guatemala—with the blatantly racist notion that indigeneity was at odds with modernity and violent efforts to eradicate it. Indigenous women's bodies became and have remained the battleground on which the fight for power in Guatemala is waged.

Global health and development programs intended to improve the health of Indigenous communities and even to empower women can play into the tropes of Maya women being non-agentive, passive recipients waiting for a solution. Many global health programs only see Maya adolescent girls and women as potential mothers rather than autonomous individuals with health needs and goals of their own, exclusively targeting them as (re)producers of children.[59] Such programs fail on multiple fronts. First, they presume to understand Maya women's goals, framing them as both monolithic and conveniently measurable via program evaluation. Second, they ignore existing community activities and leadership that women undertake. Third, they often neglect the decision-making patterns within Indigenous families and communities, which that mean adolescent girls and women's choices about their educational pathways and reproductive lives may not viewed as fully their own to make.[60]

Finally, global health systems have long relied on the unpaid labor of community health workers, and women are less likely than their male peers to be paid for this work.[61] I have been guilty of this. Our received wisdom in global health is that community participation improves programs. This is true, but all community participation is not created equal—it can meaningfully prioritize local goals and participants, or it can take advantage of local participants in service of externally defined ends. The wonderfully talented Rosi who we met at the start of the chapter was an eager participant in the group of women health promoters, but the project benefited unfairly from her talents that were only minimally compensated. For my (tiny) part, I will no longer work on global health projects that rely on volunteer labor, and I hope we are seeing the beginning of a movement in global health to fairly compensate all workers.[62] Still, global health remains a field led by men and delivered by women.[63] Women have lower-status jobs and are paid less for the same jobs as men.[64] Efforts like the Women in Global Health movement are working to draw attention to these inequalities that should be outrageous in a field committed to health equity but have gone unrecognized for too long—another underbelly of global health.

Conclusion

Global health structures and programs see themselves as empowering women, but they often collude with systems of social inequality to achieve their own self-determined, measurable outcomes. This happens from the global level to the local level. In Guatemala, women face the burden of blame for poor the health outcomes of their children, even though their choices to implement the messages of global health programs are limited by violent social structures that keep them from full public participation. Women experience social suffering as they navigate caregiving for their children and bear the sicknesses and loss of children within their homes and communities. But they also build social capital as they support one another in caregiving and agentively choose when and how to engage in treatment-seeking. Social capital is the kind of wealth that women routinely build, though for rural Maya women, it can only open some doors within Guatemala's fragmented neoliberal health care landscape. Chapter 3 explores the government health system in Guatemala and the racialized and gendered dynamics of accessing that system.

3   Of Machetes and Medicine: Troubled Pathways to Government Health Services

Doctors come when they have to come out here, but they go as soon as they can. No one stays for long. We get [medical] students, and it is just a requirement for them. This is not their place, so they go back to the city.
—community leader, a village of Acatenango

The people out in the villages don't listen, and they don't learn. They want to be left alone and keep things the way they are.
—doctor in Comalapa

I clutched my clipboard of surveys to my chest as we ran. Shouts in Kaqchikel unequivocally told us to "get off my property" after the sheet metal gate had been slammed shut in our faces. As one of the mobile doctors called in Kaqchikel through the gate, trying to convince the family inside to come out for their vaccinations, a ferociously barking dog bounded toward us from the back of the house. "Run to the truck!" one of the team shouted, and we all scrambled down the steep, rocky path to the dirt road where we had parked. Just as we were reaching the Ministry of Health truck, from somewhere up on a knoll behind a cluster of trees, came the *whirr-thump*, *whirr-thump* of small stones being hurled our way. I looked up to see a group of three or four young boys laughing as they bombarded us with debris.

We hopped into the truck and drove away as quickly as the twisting, rutted road would allow. Once back to the paved road, Carlos, one of the mobile nurses, pulled over; by then, all four of us were laughing and already retelling the story to each other of what we had seen and what we were thinking as we ran. "I told you not to try to drive up there; they don't want us up there," said Delia, a Kaqchikel nurse, still out of breath. While the rest of the group

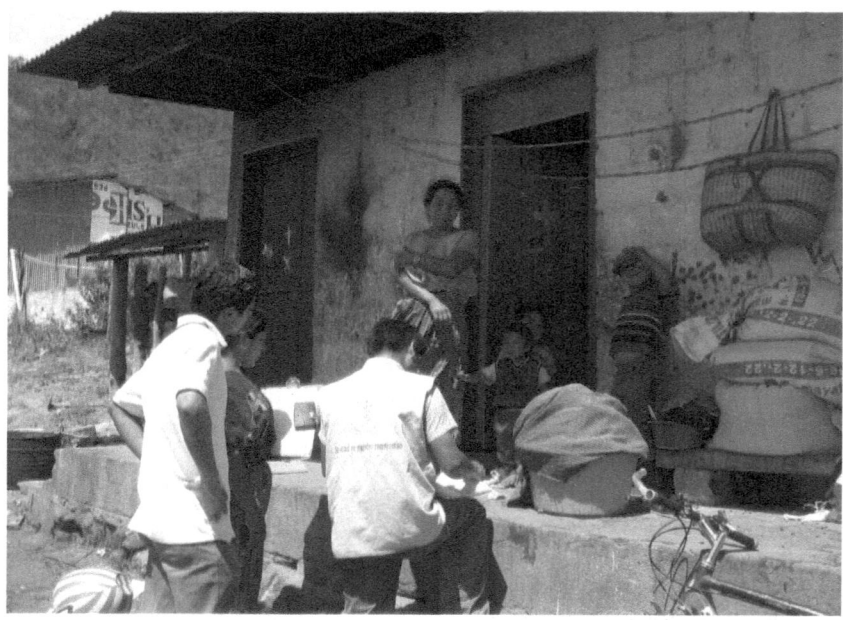

Figure 3.1
Mobile health team visiting households for vaccinations

nodded in agreement, she started marking down who the team had vaccinated and who they would not be able to reach. By this point, I had been traveling with the Acatenango mobile health team for about a month, taking surveys and talking with mothers as they waited to see the doctor. Several times people had closed their doors on us or gone to hide inside when they saw the Ministry of Health truck approaching. Still others simply smiled and refused any routine vaccinations and checkups for their children.

While there was no real danger posed by the dog and stones, it was enough to get the blood rushing, and the experience emphatically illustrated how fraught interactions with the government health system are for some of Chimaltenango's rural Maya communities. The goal of the mobile teams is to offer basic prenatal care, provide routine vaccinations and checkups for children under three, and treat or refer patients with health problems during monthly visits to each community (figure 3.1). However, as this story illustrates, some members of rural Maya communities see the mobile teams as interlopers, and interactions with the teams can be rife with suspicion, fear, and misinterpretation on all sides.

In this chapter, I explore the pluralistic care-seeking landscape for poor, rural Maya communities. I describe the Guatemalan health system as a rational structure planned to enable delivery of the human right to health but thwarted by neoliberal entanglements, weak governance, and the broader social forces of structural violence. From the bottom of the pyramid, knowledge of how to gain access to the health system is confused by an ever-changing array of services and programs that appear and disappear for many in rural Maya communities in Guatemala. We will see that marginalized populations with few economic resources face a neoliberal health system in which they recognize that better treatments and services are available but are not within their reach. Choice seems like freedom from government intrusion, but the limited choices accessible to Maya populations are shaped by deep historic and contemporary inequalities.

In this chapter, we will see how multivalent violence limits health system access for rural Maya communities. We will also see how health workers tell their own "war stories" of being chased by villagers with machetes and how they approach rural households with rocks in their fists to safeguard against guard dogs that are sometimes turned against them. Frontline health workers are given the unenviable job of bridging impossible gaps in resources and needs. Difficulties in accessing care, including the distance to facilities and the costs of supplies that should be free, lead to delays in treatment-seeking within rural Maya communities. These delays cause them to be blamed for their own poor health outcomes. Compounding challenges of care-seeking, the inadequate funding of the health system leads to seepage of staff and supplies from the government system to the private sector, and a lack of accountability leads to corruption. Using a framework of structural violence, I explore how the Guatemalan government health system generates and perpetuates predictable patterns of social suffering. Systems, structures, and programs that support, tacitly or explicitly, social inequalities are a part of the underbelly of global health.

Health Seeking within Structures of Violence

By examining rural Maya attitudes toward the health system, we can begin to understand the lasting ways in which physical violence begets and sustains structural violence within a fragmented society. While contemporary Guatemalan society is built on the violent systems of oppression established during conquest and colonization, the genocide spanning the latter half of the twentieth century viscerally imposed a social order of inequity. During the internal armed conflict, Maya community health and development workers were targeted by government-backed paramilitary groups and killed.[1] Thus, the delivery of health services is fraught with the memory of government violence against Maya communities and a refusal to allow self-determined health and development efforts. Government health services are often difficult to access, and encounters within the system are frequently marred by racism, so Maya people often choose to avoid them. The low usage rates of the health system are then pointed to by government administrators as a rational basis for limiting the expansion of government health services.

The violent marginalization enforced during wartime continues to shape peacetime realities. Rates of physical violence remain high, while structural violence continues to exclude Maya populations from social participation and access to social goods, such as health care. Indeed, participation in civil society is a risk factor for violence, and rebuilding postwar social participation amid ongoing violence has been challenging.[2] Public spaces, including health facilities, are fraught with violence—physical, symbolic, and structural. Of the all-pervasive effects of structural violence, Paul Farmer argued, "Structural violence is structured and *structuring*. It constricts the agency of its victims."[3] Structural violence works to maintain the homeostasis of injustice in society, producing and perpetuating inequalities for some and maintaining unearned advantages for others. If structural violence is the disease plaguing the Guatemalan health system, fear is its vector. Fear keeps village doors barricaded against outsiders and rocks in the wary hands of health workers. Fear, seeded by the brutal violence of the war, has shaped public engagement, trust, and community.[4] Ultimately, fear—and the legacy of physical violence on which it is based—keeps children hungry, sicknesses untreated, and Maya populations unable to fully participate and advance in Guatemalan society. In this context, the human right to health is made only of paper, far flimsier than the *piñatas* that swing from the rafters of Guatemalan markets.

The Guatemalan Health System

On paper, the Constitution of Guatemala affirms the human right to health, and the 1997 Health Code requires the Ministry of Health to provide free health care to all citizens. Yet the Guatemalan Ministry of Health is ill-equipped to address entrenched ethnic inequalities in access to health care, and its budget and political pull are weak in comparison to other government ministries. Moreover, there is a deep chasm between what has been thoughtfully planned and what actually happens in the Guatemalan health system. It is into this chasm that poor, sick, and Indigenous people fall. Here I explore the structure of the Guatemalan health system in order to understand its vulnerability to the forces of racism, corruption, and the status quo that pushes poor and Indigenous communities toward the worst health outcomes.

Health sector spending in Guatemala is 6.3 percent of gross domestic product (GDP), which is about average for Central America. However, 4 percent of GDP spending is on private, out-of-pocket health care costs by citizens. The Guatemalan government allocates only one percent of the GDP to finance the primary government health system (Ministerio de Salud Pública y Asistencia Social or MSPAS) that provides health services for 83 percent of the population. Compare this to the US government, which does not finance universal health coverage but still spends 18.3 percent of GDP on health services.[5] It is simply impossible to meet the provisions of the human right to health—available, accessible, acceptable, and high-quality services—with the resources available to the Guatemalan Ministry of Health. A series of post-conflict health sector reforms established the current national structures, and user fees were formally abolished with the 2008 Health Code to increase health system access. Yet, on-the-ground implementation of changes that would increase basic health coverage and quality has been inconsistent and incremental.

The available data echo the experiences of Rosario and her failed efforts to receive quality care for baby Efraín in Panaj and so many others in rural Maya communities across Guatemala. The 2014 Guatemala National Survey on Conditions of Life (Encuesta Nacional de Condiciones de Vida or ENCOVI) indicated that 40 percent of the population sought biomedical care for illness, accident, or preventive care; however, racial disparities persist with 47 percent of the non-Indigenous population receiving biomedical care in comparison to only 29 percent of the Indigenous population.[6] Guatemala continues to have a significant rural population, with just under 50 percent of the living in rural areas; these areas have a higher percentage of Indigenous populations. Nearly half of Guatemalans report traveling by foot to seek health care, and rural populations often must travel distances over five kilometers to the nearest health facility.[7] The landscape and infrastructure of health facilities and resources place rural residents at a distinct disadvantage for seeking timely, appropriate health services.

The government health infrastructure in Guatemala consists of a tiered system of facilities ranging from local health posts up to tertiary care hospitals (see figure 3.2). To serve a population of 17 million, the government health system has forty-three hospitals: seventeen at the department level, ten at the district level, seven at the regional level, six specialized facilities, and three general hospitals that take referrals. The specialized and general hospitals are clustered in the Guatemala City area. In addition to the hospitals, there are 279 health centers, 903 health posts, and forty-six enhanced health posts.[8] Health centers are divided into Type A and B facilities, with Type A facilities able to provide inpatient care and most often found in large urban areas. Since 2015, the government has prioritized convergence

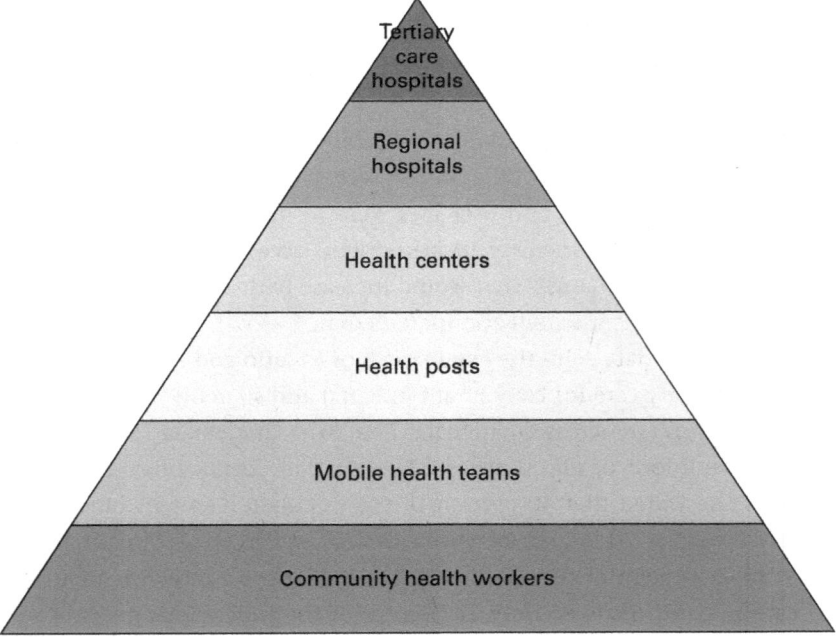

Figure 3.2
Guatemalan government health system structure.

centers (*centros de convergencia*) to support ambulatory health teams in communities without a dedicated health facility. Guatemala also has a national system of social security, the Guatemalan Social Security Institute (IGSS), through which people who work in formal employment sectors can qualify for health coverage. IGSS insures only about 17 percent of the population but has a parallel structure of hospitals and health posts.[9] Just as health facilities are heavily weighted toward urban areas, the distribution of health workers favors urban areas: 25.7 health workers per 10,000 population in urban areas in comparison to only 3.0 per 10,000 in rural areas.[10]

Rural Maya communities in Chimaltenango and across Guatemala are undergoing a quiet crisis of primary health care. Community health workers (CHWs) have formed the local face of primary care in communities since the 1970s, variously supported through different models and programs by both the government and nongovernmental organizations (NGOs).[11] In Guatemala, CHWs capture a heterogeneous group of local community members variously trained to provide health education, triage basic health concerns, and collect epidemiologic data.[12] The once-promising system of CHWs has eroded, yet new comprehensive, basic health care services have been slow to take root in their stead. Mobile health teams are met with mixed responses from the populations they serve, and even if they were welcomed by all, they could not meet the human right to health with a monthly visit to communities and only basic supplies. Rural and ethnic differences in access to the formal health system become the paramount issue in determining successes in utilization of oral rehydration therapy (ORT) and in triaging more severe cases of diarrhea in a timely manner.

A 2003 study conducted by the Guatemalan Association of Community Health Services (ASECSA) estimated use of the government health services at 35 percent in Indigenous populations; however, the study also found that referrals to CHWs from local healers were a common occurrence.[13] In my own survey, 72 percent of Maya respondents reported that they would acquire treatment for sick children at a government health facility, either a health post or center or the departmental hospital. Yet in-depth interview and focus-group data lead me to believe my survey results obscure the position of government health services, which are often used as an option of last resort.[14] Data on health system utilization show persistent challenges in reaching racial and geographic parity in health system access, though the intercultural unit of the MSPAS has had some modest successes, such as having facilities to support traditional birth positions in about half of the health centers. Maya communities have relatively high use rates for government childhood vaccination programs, but there are larger disparities across other health services, such as contraception and care for chronic conditions for which private-sector services are more commonly used.[15]

Tiers of the Health System in Chimaltenango

As the departmental capital, Chimaltenango has a hospital that receives referrals from municipal health centers throughout the department (figure 3.3). A clinic attached to the hospital serves as the local health center for cases that do not require the hospital's more advanced services. The hospital itself includes an emergency room, pediatric ward, adult ward, two operating rooms, a two-story maternal care unit, a laboratory, and X-ray room.[16] With these facilities, the government hospital is the most well-equipped and provides the highest level of care available in the department. Public facilities as

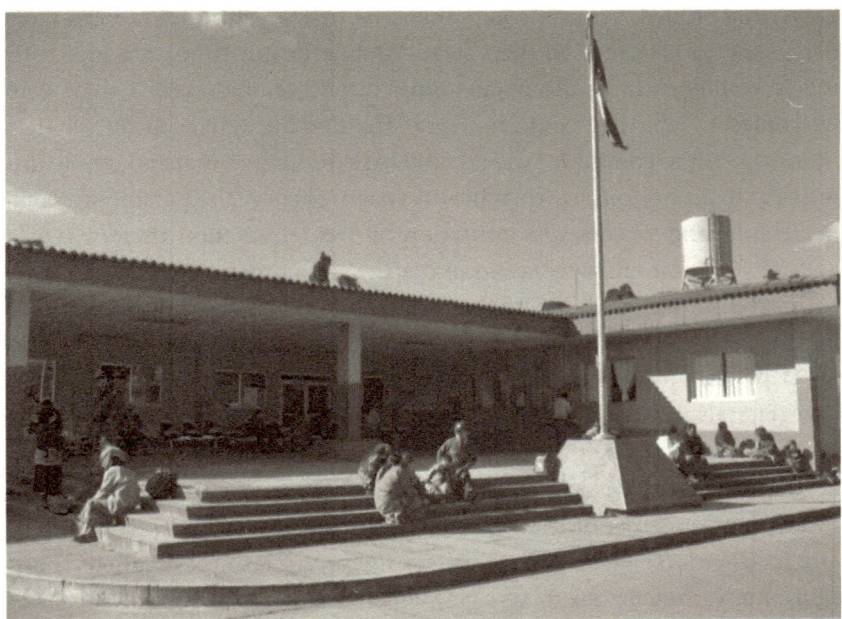

Figure 3.3
Chimaltenango Departmental Hospital.

well as private practices refer cases that they cannot treat to the hospital. In rare instances, the hospital will refer cases, normally for advanced surgery or specialized treatments, to the appropriate tertiary care hospital in Guatemala City.

Doctors and nursing staff at the Chimaltenango Hospital reported in interviews that delayed arrival of patients from outlying communities was a significant barrier to the provision of effective care. They commented that doctors out in the municipal health centers often wait too long, thinking that they can treat a patient at their own facility rather than immediately referring them to the hospital. Patients' reluctance and inability to travel to the hospital, since there is no standard ambulance service outside of the city of Chimaltenango, means that they often delay the trip to the hospital until the situation is extremely dire. Services at the hospital are free, though a patient must pay for lab tests, X-rays, and consumable supplies such as needles.

The hospital staff report that delayed admission makes their case-fatality ratios look unfairly poor, and patients are reluctant to come to a facility they associate with high mortality rates. Hospital doctors further reported that they receive several cases each week from private doctors and clinics where cases have become too complicated for the private facilities to handle. I saw this occur in at least two cases during my long-term fieldwork in 2006 and 2007, when surgical cases from NGO and private clinics were sent on to the government hospital in which the referred patients ultimately died. This is a phenomenon I have continued to observe in short-term medical missions of foreign health providers.[17]

Government hospitals do see patients with the most dire, emergent conditions that all too often have bad outcomes, so perhaps the negative reputation they have, particularly among Indigenous communities, is unfair. Yet the broader health system and human context in which hospitals are embedded funnel people toward outcomes that seem predetermined. Symbolic violence makes individuals within a system acquiesce to structural violence—of course, the rural, Indigenous poor expect bad outcomes in hospitals just as rich, urban ladinos expect good ones. This is understood as the natural order of things. Except, of course this is a fallacy.[18] Poor health systems outcomes are patterned by wealth and race by human-design, not some inherent rule of the cosmos. Delays in treatment-seeking due to structural barriers, such as distance and ancillary costs, and the difficult-to-tabulate social barriers of racism and social exclusion lead to the poorer outcomes for Maya people in Guatemala's hospitals.

While hospitals form the apex of the health system, treatment-seeking often begins in a lower-level facility. The next level down in the government health care hierarchy is the municipal health centers. Both Acatenango and Comalapa serve as municipal seats and, consequently, have health centers. With a smaller population, Acatenango has a smaller type B health center, while Comalapa has a larger type A health center. However, both have essentially the same facilities: two exam/patient rooms, nurse's room, laboratory, drug storage area, and offices. Although Comalapa's health center (figure 3.4) is classified as type A, it does not typically have the staff to treat patients overnight, and it provides the same basic services as the smaller Acatenango center. The primary difference in patient service between the two facilities is that the Comalapa center is staffed by a doctor each weekday through the afternoon and the Acatenango center only has a doctor present during four weekday mornings.

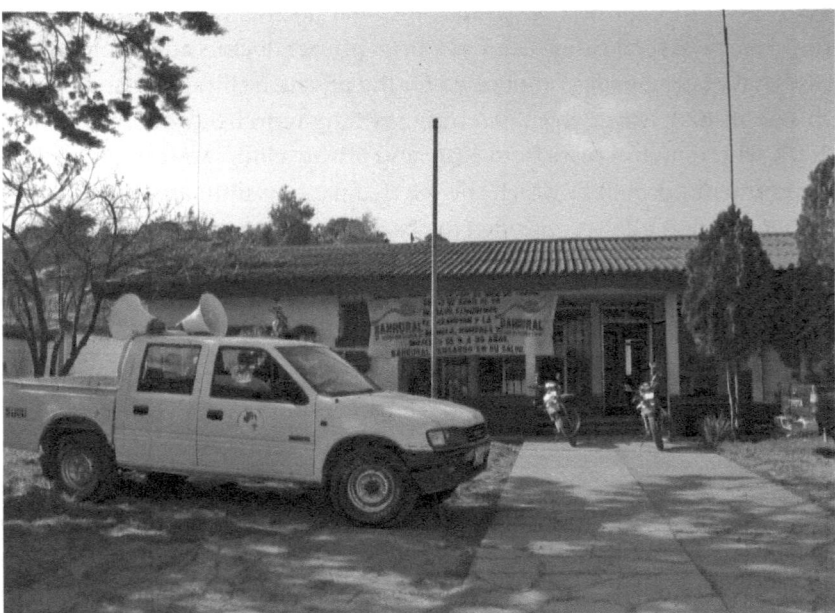

Figure 3.4
Comalapa Health Center.

In addition to having doctors on staff, health centers coordinate and implement national health initiatives for their municipalities, such as vaccination campaigns. To reach the entire population of a municipality, health centers coordinate with mobile health teams who travel monthly to all communities in the municipality. The teams, which typically consist of a doctor and two or more nurses, work with local community health workers to hold clinic hours, provide vaccinations, and distribute nutritional supplements for lactating mothers and children under two. These services vary depending on national political will and the whims of international aid funding.

Local health posts and convergence centers that host mobile teams serve as the primary level of health care for rural residents. Health posts are distributed throughout municipalities in the larger communities. The health posts across Chimaltenango, as in the rest of the country, vary immensely in the type of facilities, services offered, and hours of operation. As an example of the best equipped facilities, the health post in one peri-urban village of Acatenango had its own building, which was built by the community. The facility has a main waiting area with four rooms leading from it: an exam room, medicine storage room, the doctor's office, and a room with a bed if someone needs to stay overnight, though this is extremely rare. This post is staffed on weekday mornings by a medical student from Guatemala City.

However, most health posts consist of a dedicated room in a community health worker's house, often without electricity or flooring (figure 3.5). The room typically has a table for patient exams and a locked cupboard for medicine storage. Most health posts are staffed only by CHWs, most often men from the local community, who help publicize when the mobile teams will be coming to hold a clinic day. In communities where there is no health post, the mobile teams operate out of convergence centers or pickup trucks. When a community health worker manages a health post and regularly sees patients, they are supposed to be compensated monthly. A lower tier of CHWs, often referred to as health promoters (though this term is sometimes used for fee-for-service private providers), is made up of volunteers who share public health education messages within their communities and refer people to care. Health promoters are given only a small incentive for participation and are more often women in comparison to CHWs. The quality and amount of training and oversight for health promoters varies significantly across municipalities. Remember that the health promoter group that we met in chapter 1 pushed back against an ORT curriculum that did not make

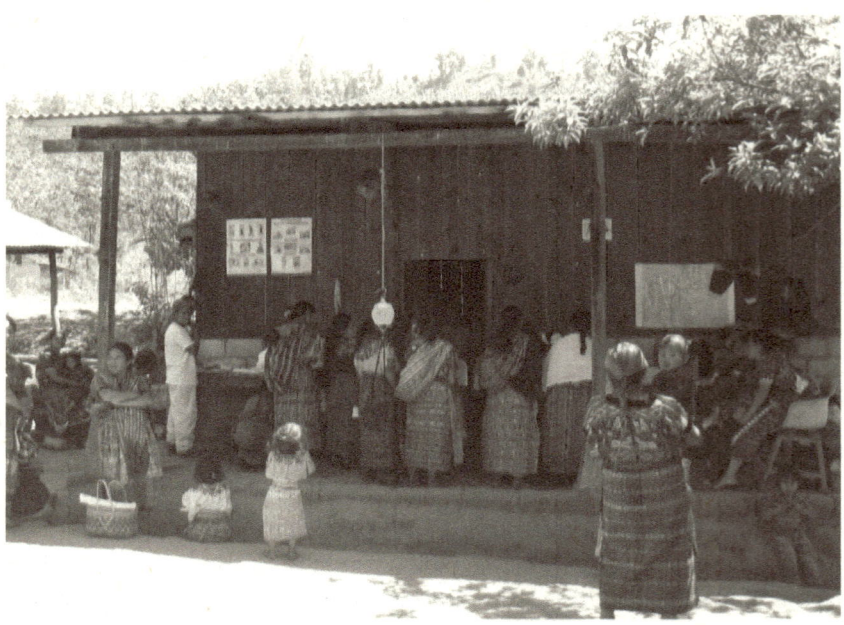

Figure 3.5
Health post in a village near Comalapa.

sense for their community. In reality, health promoters are rarely given the opportunity to shape programs or fully harness their local expertise in delivering programs developed in Guatemala City and often before that in global health and development hubs like Geneva and Washington, DC.

Neoliberal Reforms and the Bottom of the Pyramid

Structural violence is multivalent. Just as the structure of the health system benefits urban elites and disenfranchises the rural poor, foreign aid comes on the terms set by high-income countries. The foreign aid and development packages offered to Guatemala by multilateral organizations and high-income country governments to rebuild society following the internal armed conflict required the state to implement cost-cutting and privatized neoliberal approaches to public systems from agrarian reform to security (or perceptions of it) to the health care landscape.[19] The "success" of the peace process was defined as a reinvigorated neoliberal approach and improved economic indicators, with an infusion of wealth cascading across sectors and social schisms to rebuild society.[20] Salmaan Keshavjee has described "neoliberal programmatic blindness" in which funding programs determine the type of global health and development programming delivered, even if it is not the best fit for the context.[21] The financial superstructure of global health and development perpetrates structural violence, furnishing gifts with strings attached that tie systems to particular approaches and maintain global power asymmetries. Just as the rural Maya are positioned as supplicants on the fringes of the health system, the Guatemalan government is positioned as a supplicant to the global health polity.

The 1996 Peace Accords established the Integrated System of Health Attention (SIAS for the Spanish acronym) as a mechanism for creating a primary care structure that could rapidly provide coverage across the distinct geographic and cultural regions of Guatemala. Through the extension of coverage program, SIAS set up a system in which nongovernmental organizations were contracted by the government to provide primary care for a specific region, usually operating at the municipal level. The NGOs were responsible for the hiring, training, and management of the mobile health teams that served rural communities and those without staffed health facilities. The NGOs were also responsible for the instruction of CHWs. The public-private partnerships (formal relationships established between state and nonstate actors) established through SIAS reflected neoliberal development trends toward decentralization and the encouragement of civil participation.[22] Yet, SIAS restricted partner NGOs to administrative roles functioning within the traditional health system structure, which limited their ability to adapt programs and delivery of care to local contexts and undermined the goals of decentralization.[23]

In 2012, the Guatemalan government estimated that SIAS was providing health and nutrition services to 54 percent of the rural population.[24] Despite being the vanguard of health services for a large segment of the population, SIAS was vulnerable to the political priorities of each presidential administration and weakened by poor financing. Ironically, SIAS partner NGOs introduced planning and monitoring into the primary health system, yet the impacts of SIAS as a health sector strategy were not thoroughly evaluated.[25] Reforms were made to SIAS to expand programming and the use of convergence centers in 2012, but critiques about lack of oversight and corruption within the system grew, and arguments that the decentralized program was more costly than traditional direct service delivery emerged. In 2013, a law was passed that forbid the government to contract out service delivery to nonstate actors.[26] Payment to SIAS partner NGOs was abruptly halted in 2014, despite plans for phased change.[27] Rural areas experienced health facility closures, stoppages of services, and staff who worked without pay for up to eighteen months. Plans for government-delivered primary health care were implemented rapidly and continue to be refined. The low availability of health workers in rural areas meant that most of the same providers who worked through SIAS are now working directly through the government. The frustration of frontline health providers was understandable, as they picked up the slack for the gap in functioning government primary care programs within communities.

In an added layer of complexity, pharmaceuticals are supplied through a system of public and private pharmacies. Drugs distributed in Guatemala are manufactured in eighty-five national and two foreign laboratories. In 1999, government drug spending was approximately US$17 million, and private spending was approximately US$130 million. A 1997 agreement for the joint negotiation of drug purchase prices by the Ministry of Public Health, IGSS, and the military medical service was intended to keep prices in government pharmacies low.[28] However, prices tend to be comparable to privately owned pharmacies. Legally, Guatemalan pharmacies must be overseen by a trained pharmacist, yet most operate as informal shops with no one trained in pharmaceuticals present. Many medications controlled in high-income countries, such as antibiotics, are available over-the-counter in Guatemala. Although efforts have been made to control the distribution of antibiotics, essentially narcotics are the only class of drug that is tightly controlled.

Patient Perspectives on Health-Seeking through Structures of Violence

Ana, Flavia's neighbor in Panaj, was a young Kaqchikel Maya mother pregnant with her third baby in three years. She was soft-spoken and mostly kept inside her household, tending her little ones and doing household chores with her mother-in-law. She had left school after three years to work in her father's fields on a slope overlooking the village, and she told me once that she was too shy to join the local women's weaving cooperative because she was unsure she could follow the intricate patterns on her loom. Despite her shyness, Ana always went out to see the mobile health teams when they came to the village. One morning, I sat out at the crossroad in the center of the village chatting with women as they waited for their turn with the health team. After a long wait, Ana's name was called, and she popped up anxiously to take her turn. Before she could even reach the dropped tailgate of the truck that formed the consultation desk, the ladino doctor boomed, "Whoa, are you pregnant again? Incredible! You people just keep going," and he raised his eyebrows suggestively. Ana froze, and the other women giggled nervously. Ana proceeded to get prenatal vitamins and nutritional supplements for her two children, quietly answering the health team's questions in as few words as possible. I caught up to her as she walked home and asked if she was okay. "Yes," she said, "It's embarrassing, but everybody knows he's [the doctor] like that. I know my kids need the vitamins to make sure they grow strong."

As Ana's story and those of so many others illustrate, health-seeking is an act of bravery and optimism in Guatemala if you are poor and Maya. It requires bravery knowing that you may be subjected to discrimination and further harmed by the institutions that are meant to heal. It requires optimism that the social structures that circumscribe your life will somehow be different this time and include you as a person worthy of care. Barbara Rylko-Bauer, Linda Whiteford, and Paul Farmer enumerate an important list of the impacts of violence on health-seeking, including issues from the disruption of families and communities of support through stress and the long-term embodied impacts of trauma.[29] To their list of nine items, I would add another: generations of violence makes violence culturally acceptable and expected, creating populations inured to violence and setting in motion future chains of acquiescence. The centuries of violent repression from the time of conquest and the heightened violence of the Guatemalan internal armed conflict have left little hope for Indigenous populations that they are entitled to and can expect to receive social goods, such as the human right to health guaranteed to them in the 1996 Peace Accords. They expect, to the contrary, what they have received for generations—inferior positions within societal structures violently stacked against them. Within this system, they must make choices on how to best care for their families and how to survive.

Routine health-seeking for children primarily falls to women in rural Maya communities. In large part this is because caregiving for children is considered women's work, but it is also because of the paternalistic way that health care is delivered (see figure 3.6). The often-demeaning way that

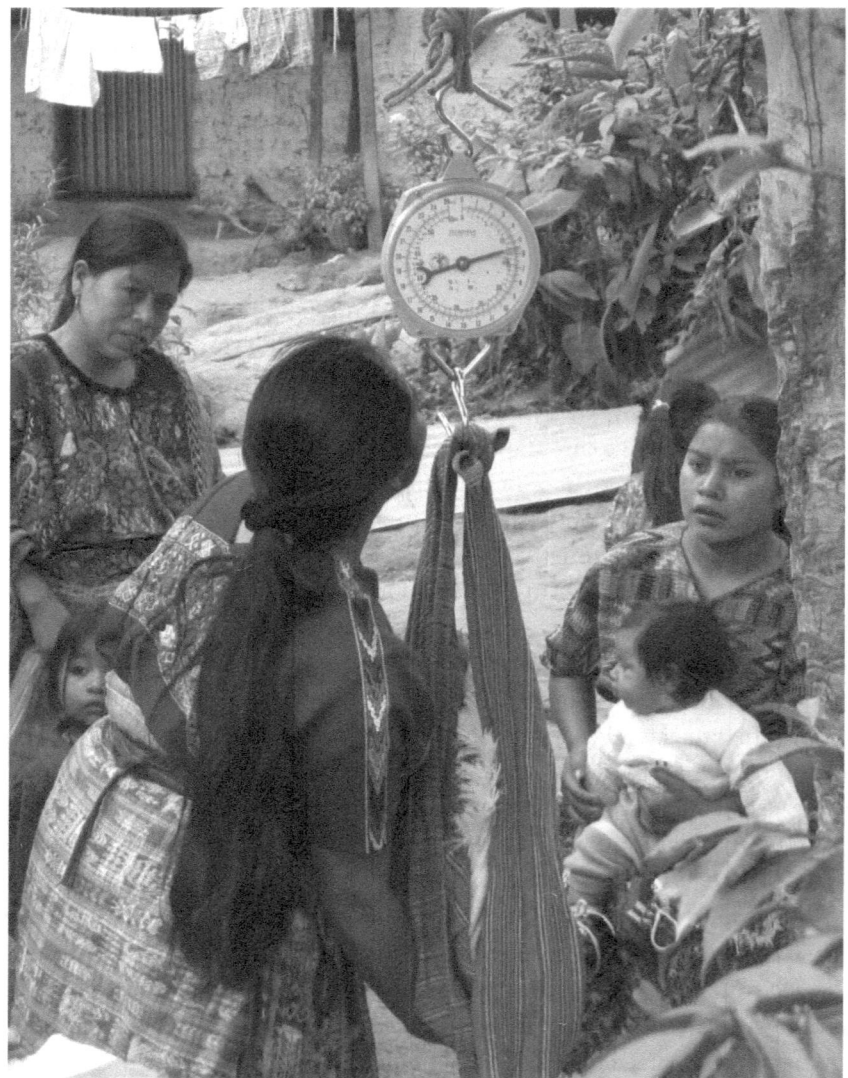

Figure 3.6
Community health promoters weigh a baby in a village near Comalapa.

patient-provider interactions are structured is more likely to be tolerated by women. In my observation, the mobile team (male) doctors consistently spoke to rural Maya care-seekers in slow, loud, imperative statements. I often watched one of the two Comalapa mobile health teams say to mothers in loud, frustrated tones, "*Digo yo . . .*" or "I say . . ." that you have to do this or that. In all patient-provider interactions that I observed, there was a distinct one-sidedness to the conversations and never a dialogue. The doctors believe that they have the answers for how mothers can best achieve health for their children, and the hierarchical structure of Guatemalan society means that Maya women feel they cannot question a doctor's methods or treatment, even when they do not fully understand what they are being told to do. In exchanges with patients and parents, mobile doctors come across at best as paternalistic and at worse as dictatorial.

Many Maya men are distrustful of the mobile health teams and their motivations and sometimes tell their wives to stay away from them when they make their monthly rounds. When I was living in Panaj, I found that my good friend Juana stayed inside her house with the door closed and kept her children with her when she heard the health team coming. This behavior was entirely out of character for Juana, whom I knew to be talkative and sociable and who typically kept her door open to the sunlight as she worked around the house all day. During one of their visits, I greeted the mobile team who I knew from having worked with them previously, and I talked with other villagers as they came to the truck parked at the village crossroads to have consultations and receive powdered nutritional supplements. I even went with the mobile team as they walked through the village to find children needing vaccinations that had not been brought out to see them. At one point, we stood outside Juana's house as one of the nurses knocked and called out to her. I knew she was inside but, of course, did not say anything, and the team gave up and went on to the next child on their list.

Later, after the health truck had left in a cloud of dust headed back to Comalapa, I went back by Juana's house. The door was once again flung open, and she was bustling about her yard chopping firewood and beginning preparations for lunch. When she saw me, she started giggling, saying, "I figured you were probably with them earlier." I said that I had been, but that it was her business whether she wanted to use the health service or not. "It's my husband," she said. "He says it's best if we stay off of all the lists.

We don't want them [the government] to know everything about where we are and what we do. It's safest to keep to ourselves." This attitude toward the health service, and the government more generally, reflects the continued distrust instilled in the Indigenous population during the years of the internal armed conflict. Juana's brother-in-law and two of her cousins were killed during the violence, though she vehemently says that none of them were involved on either the army or guerrilla groups. We can see from Juana's example that suspicion and fear of the government are still critical issues that hinder particularly the rural Indigenous population from fully and comfortably using even minimal government health services. Juana told me that she has seen the mobile doctor before and that she took her three-year-old son to the health center in Comalapa once when he broke his arm. She rated the service as "okay" but still said that she did not like having to see the doctors and that she waits to see if it is something very serious before she considers using the health system.

Despite the derision, unease, or embarrassment they may face in engaging with government health services, most Maya mothers say they think that biomedicine is the best way to heal a sick child. Over and over again, I heard village women say in focus-group discussions that, if given unlimited money to use to improve childhood diarrhea in their communities, they would pay to have a doctor in the village or, from those who were unable to even conceive of this flight of imagination, that they would pay for a truck to take sick children to the health center in town. Therefore, women's willingness and, as in Juana's case, their permission to interact with health staff is heavily contingent on their financial resources and tempered by the setting in which health care is delivered.

Where some women appreciated the convenience of health staff being in their village monthly, most responded negatively when the mobile teams made surprise "house calls," which removes choice from their health-seeking actions. The default response to unplanned visits was suspicion and closed doors. Upon arriving in a village, one of the Comalapa mobile teams sometimes drove around the surrounding area announcing their visit through a public-address system installed in their truck. While admittedly this gave those who did not want to be seen for vaccinations a chance to hide, I found that most people responded well to this approach. Women could have the opportunity to stop their work and gather their children before coming to a central point in the village to see the mobile team. This way they did not have to have health staff, who are viewed as government agents, coming onto their property and into their homes. I believe this is a positive approach toward reducing some of the tension surrounding the health team visits and more closely replicates the services for people living in towns with health centers in that they can approach the health service on their own terms in a centralized location.

While living in rural villages for many months, I observed that women are far more likely to consult with a CHW when that individual is already well known to them either through friendship or kinship ties. When the CHW is less known to a mother seeking treatment for a child with diarrhea, she is less likely to have a consultation within the first forty-eight hours of the onset of the child's illness, and this time lag increases to between two and four days if there is no one acting as a community health worker in the location of residence. Further, mothers are far less likely to adequately learn how to administer ORT correctly if they do not have an existing close relationship with the community health worker. This seems to be because women do not want to ask questions when ORT is explained or make a return visit to ask follow-up questions to someone not well known to them.

Even when caregivers navigate the system and seek care, the quality of care received can be poor, and outcomes from programming short-lived or even harmful. My friend Estrella, mother of three young children in Panaj, explained to me her knowledge of ORT: "They [CHWs] tell us it's good, and we use it. And it's good. It stops the sickness—dries them [the children with diarrhea] up. There's no more diarrhea if you give ORT." Of the women who reported knowing about ORT in my in-depth interviews and focus-group discussions, only about 10 percent were able to describe an effective preparation and administration of an oral rehydration salts solution. Even of those mothers who could describe to me step-by-step how they would use ORT, all but a very few expressed unrealistic expectations of the outcomes that ORT would deliver—namely, that it would stop the diarrhea. This idea was in many instances supported by CHWs and even mobile team staff, sometimes out of zeal in promoting ORT or a lack of knowledge themselves. The number and level of involvement of community health workers is extremely varied by village, as is their level of knowledge on basic treatments for childhood illnesses, including ORT.

While engagement with mobile teams and travel to health posts and centers can be challenging, navigating inpatient, facility-based care for children with diarrhea brings distinct concerns. I interviewed twenty-five mothers in the government hospital and two mothers at a private hospital whose children had been admitted for inpatient care due to diarrhea. Most of the children experienced moderate to severe levels of dehydration, which prompted their admittance for intravenous (IV) fluids. In the government hospital, a designated pediatric rehydration ward was set up during the rotavirus season from November to February. The ethnicity of inpatients was equally split between ladino and Kaqchikel Maya. However, ladino patients were far more likely to live in the urban and peri-urban areas of Chimaltenango and to have experienced the current bout of diarrhea for only an average of two days before being brought to the hospital.[30] Kaqchikel patients, on the other hand, had more often traveled in from rural towns and villages, with travel time ranging from thirty minutes to three hours. They had been sick an average of ten days prior to being brought to a hospital for treatment.[31]

Mothers at the government hospital were very pleased with the care their children were receiving. They spoke of the IV fluids as "miraculous" and "the only treatment that really works." One Maya mother who had traveled three hours with her two-year-old daughter to the hospital said, "You know, it is a relief to be here. It means that the doctor is responsible and that my daughter will be better." We can see that this mother, like the other women I spoke with on the rotavirus ward, had faith in the treatment that her child would receive. Further, she felt that a burden of responsibility had been lifted off her shoulders by doing everything she could by bringing her child to the hospital. The mothers I interviewed, both in the hospital and other contexts, believed that hospital care was the best possible treatment for children with what they deemed severe diarrhea.

Provider Perspectives of Healing within Systems of Violence

It is tempting to blame health providers for their roles in systems that perpetuate violent marginalization. But there are few bad actors among them. As individuals, they want to do their jobs. They want to help people be healthy. They work within a health system that is underfunded, with little support or training in how to engage with the rural poor much less how to enact health equity. "They really do not like being bothered by the health team in these [rural] communities, particularly for mandatory vaccinations.

We have been met with violence in the past and have been threatened with machetes," recounted a mobile doctor in Comalapa. Inasmuch as Indigenous patients and community members are wary of government health workers, the health workers often perceive their job as dangerous, saying that it takes people of great courage and determination to do what they do. Government health workers have huge administrative burdens and provider-patient ratios beyond the possibility of mortals to fulfill. They often work multiple jobs because of low pay in the public sector.

I rode along with mobile health teams in Acatenango and Comalapa and observed the doctors and nurses interacting with patients. Over the course of my time with the teams, I had the opportunity to have extensive conversations with the teams about their work and their perceptions of the patients they serve. I both conducted a large focus group discussion and many informal individual interviews with community health workers. I also conducted interviews with staff at health centers and the government hospital. During these conversations, providers across multiple tiers of the government health system were able to share their views and frustrations surrounding the implementation of ORT.

Seeking to build on the limited health workforce, NGO community health workers were first integrated with the government health system in Chimaltenango in 1975. This was an effort on the part of the Ministry of Public Health to be more culturally sensitive to the health care needs and preferences of the department's Maya population.[32] However, community distrust of the government health system runs deeper than intercultural differences, despite the good intentions of providers. Though some members of the mobile teams may be from humble origins, many express disdain or even disgust for the way people in the villages live—without clean water, toilets, or tiled floors. Most of the mobile health staff express exhaustion and frustration with their jobs, and many of them are young people who will only remain in their positions until they can find a better one in an urban location.

One doctor in Comalapa was told when he was hired, "We'll see how long you last." He went on to say, "I hate that people don't want my help. They think of us as the enemy." Interestingly, he and another ambulatory doctor in Comalapa independently mentioned that it is not always the most rural populations who reject their services; rather, he pointed to informal settlements, such as those that have grown up around the edges of Comalapa, as most reluctant. The houses in these communities are illegally built on untenanted land, are typically of poor construction, and have no access to municipal utilities (i.e., electricity, water). It makes sense that these communities would resist interactions with government health employees, since they live in fear that the government will one day get around to pushing them off the land.

Thus, fear and feelings of social distance abound on both sides of health delivery. Making matters worse, many mobile health workers fail to be sensitive to the memories of wartime violence held by many in the communities they serve. One afternoon, a tired mobile team drove through communities outside Comalapa announcing a vaccination campaign for adults. Frustrated by low turnout, they took to shouting through the truck's public-address system that anyone who did not receive the vaccination would be pulled out into the street and arrested by the police. These statements were made as a joke, accompanied by laughter, but were unlikely to be interpreted in the same manner of levity by local residents who had, in fact, had family members dragged from their homes, never to be seen again.

Members of the mobile teams are in some part hired for their expressed desire to work in underserved communities and in some instances for their ability to speak Kaqchikel. However, of the seven native Kaqchikel-speaking mobile doctors and nurses with whom I worked closely in Acatenango and Comalapa, only one regularly spoke with patients in Kaqchikel. To say that the mobile teams are people of the communities they serve is a falsehood. While it may appear so on paper, these doctors and nurses, by virtue of their education and status in the wider context of Guatemalan society, are very different from their patients. To speak Kaqchikel makes some of the nurses and doctors uncomfortable—they received their medical educations in Spanish and have left behind the life and lifestyle in which they may have primarily spoken Kaqchikel. In most instances when Kaqchikel is spoken during a consultation, it is after several loud, slow attempts have been made to explain the diagnosis and treatment to the patient or caregiver in Spanish.

In a rare example of syncretism on the part of government health providers, I saw one Kaqchikel doctor tell a postpartum Maya woman in a rural village not to eat anything green, like avocado, broccoli, or cucumber, because it would be too cooling for her breastmilk and would give the baby colic. It was heartening to see the woman respond affirmatively, and she seemed open to the doctor's other postnatal instructions, including perineal care, that may have been less familiar. Providers like this one work so hard to build a bridge through a fragmented and exclusionary health system for their patients, but they are too few and up against barriers too large for individuals to dismantle alone. The health system cannot rely on a few intercultural brokers to "reach" Maya populations; indeed, even health providers from a Maya background can perpetrate cultural violence and exclusionary practices. Reliance on a veneer of interculturalism helps maintain a system that explicitly refuses to center the needs of Maya communities.

Delays in Accessing the Government Health System

Violence shapes health because people put off care-seeking due to fear of interacting with the government system, myriad accessibility barriers, and entrenched norms of racialized marginalization. Health center and hospital staff tend to see more serious cases of diarrhea, particularly from rural patients because of delayed care-seeking. Like Juana, mothers living in rural villages postpone a visit to the health center until they perceive that a condition is serious. Their reasons are the distance to facilities, the cost of getting there, and their reluctance to interact with the health system. These delays are frustrating and can cost the health and lives of children. It is so easy to look at the tiered health system, the steps so neatly laid out, and unfairly blame mothers for the delays. It is easy for government health officials to blame them for not doing what they should, for not being "rational" consumers of the services provided. Yet, we have seen the incredible challenges in care-seeking that make their delays, their wait-and-see approaches, understandable. Mothers—and fathers and grandparents and kin—make choices, often with limited information and resources, to do the best they can for their children.

The primary outcome of the many barriers to accessing health services is that treatment-seeking is delayed. The costs of health-seeking in a free government system can be a key challenge, with families losing time at work and needing to pay for travel, lab and diagnostic tests, and medical supplies. The physiological effects of diarrhea are worsened by the amount of time a child goes untreated, particularly with regard to dehydration for acute diarrhea and undernutrition for repeated bouts of diarrhea. Long-term impacts of delayed treatment-seeking for diarrhea, as in the case of a child I met in hospital who had diarrhea for forty days, can include undernutrition, prompting losses and delays in developmental milestones and growth stunting.

Figure 3.7 shows an aggregate treatment-seeking decision timeline for rural mothers. The timeline shows how they prioritize resources, relying first on treatments available close to home and, if the diarrhea continues, gradually seeking treatments that are costlier and further afield. The decision timeline differs for rural mothers compared to the one used by mothers living in towns and cities, who typically resort to a health center or hospital after two days, particularly if a case of diarrhea is deemed severe. Urban women, even if living in poverty, have fewer geographic barriers and are more likely to be participating more fully in the cash economy than their rural peers, enabling greater access health services. A notable exception to the rule that people who live further away wait longer to seek can be found in the emerging, unauthorized, peri-urban settlements on the outskirts of towns. Because of the stigma and marginal status of these communities, residents of peri-urban settlements are as unlikely as their isolated rural counterparts to access the health system, despite their relatively close proximity to health centers.

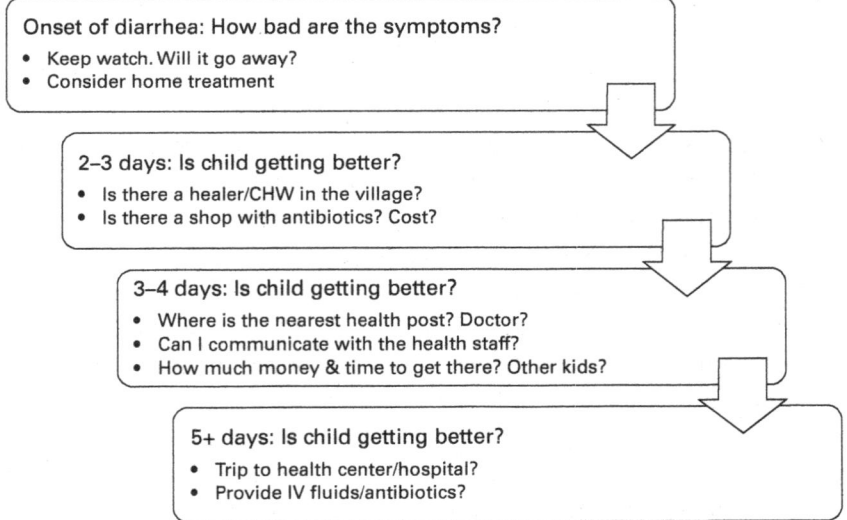

Figure 3.7
Diarrhea treatment decision timeline for rural mothers.

Waiting too long to treat childhood diarrhea can have dire consequences. A mother from a village of Acatenango told me, "I have known three children to die from diarrhea in my village. They were taken to the hospital, but they died on the way. This happens to poor families. They rely on the few medicines they are given, and when they come to the health center it is too late." The length of time a mother will wait before moving to the next option for care depends on her assessment of the severity of the diarrhea. Biomedical treatment is more often sought for childhood illness in Guatemala when the illness is perceived to be severe.[33]

Health centers have the equipment to give intravenous fluids to dehydrated children, although the director of the Comalapa health center reported that parents usually prefer to take their children to the hospital in Chimaltenango once an illness is severe. The Comalapa health center provided packets of oral rehydration salts to mothers who have children currently experiencing diarrhea. The Acatenango health post frequently experienced stockouts and instead referred mothers to pharmacies or back to their community health workers, creating a fruitless loop within the health system. Health centers have laboratory facilities where they can test stool samples to attempt to determine the causal pathogen in cases of diarrhea that do not resolve, and they give free medicines on the basis of test results. When I asked a lab technician at the Acatenango health center if there is a problem with antibiotic resistance since they only dispensed one type of antibiotic, she said that there were some cases of resistance caused by patient (caregiver) noncompliance. She added that she thought these cases would work themselves out because the child's parents could get more antibiotics in the market.

During the rotavirus season from November to February, the government hospital in Chimaltenango dedicated an entire ward to children with rotavirus. Once admitted to the ward, children, ranging in age from just a few months to four years old, were uniformly given IV fluids as a part of their treatment, usually in conjunction with acetaminophen for fever. Most children stay as inpatients from between four to eight days, depending on the severity of the case and the overall nutritional status of the child. The chief of pediatrics at the Chimaltenango government hospital told me:

> Community programs should be strengthened. If the community programs functioned better, the cases here would be less severe. The health centers really don't work; they should be [open] twenty-four hours. Patients prefer the hospital because there are staff people here all the time. All of our departments are full all the time.

He further expressed his belief that the population of Chimaltenango resists ORT and that they use herbs and other treatments to try to dry up diarrhea. They are not able to do any ORT education in the pediatric wards because there is only one nurse for every thirty children. He said he would like to have a dedicated ward for rehydration where mothers could learn from the nurses how to use ORT, but this is not possible given the overstretched hospital resources. Much like his patients and their parents, the chief of pediatrics believed that the hospital treatment that children with diarrhea receive is adequate. But, he asserted that the fault lines in the health system run through the health centers and posts, which are intended to provide primary care and prevention education. So much hard work by well-intentioned providers at every level goes into a health system that is fundamentally flawed in its resource allocation and, by proxy, its estimation of human value.

Neoliberal Oversight and Health Sector Corruption

Development is too often framed as a teleological process that happens *to* people. Health systems strengthening is defined through statistics like provider-patient ratios, no matter how the numerator or denominator may view the state of things. The vague definitions of those predetermined end points and distant benchmarks are set by outsiders, who cast local populations as passive recipients without agency. Within neoliberal development and global health models, measurable outcomes become the goal rather than real and lasting change determined by local people. The transition from previous international health and development paradigms to contemporary global health over the past thirty years reflects neoliberal values, particularly evidence-based statistics and cost-effectiveness.[34] Realities falling outside externally mandated metrics cease to exist within the worlds of global health program evaluation, government accountability mechanisms, and financial reporting.

While enumeration can mean empowerment in global health, within the Guatemalan context, statistics are fraught—the Maya population struggles to "count" within society as powerful elites manipulate the numbers of those killed by genocide and of ongoing evidence of inequities.[35] Even as we have seen significant public-private partnerships in Guatemala with NGOs in the health sector, NGOs replicate the models of government systems, with an emphasis on delivering measurable programs to show organizational self-efficacy while compelling gratitude from recipients.[36] In the name of measurability, global health programs can create relationships and categories of experience that did not exist locally solely to quantify and evaluate programs.[37] More nuanced approaches to implementing global health programs and understanding their impacts are possible. Approaches that center the agency of communities can help unpack the power dynamics within development programs and can enable health worker agency within global health programs.[38] The people who engage with systems are more than numbers—we need metrics, but we should be aware of their shortcomings and the realities they obscure by design.

A few years ago, I saw firsthand how numbers are slippery and health sector corruption can work to conceal data that do not fit preferred narratives for program outcomes. I was working with some summer students on data analysis in an office in Antigua, Guatemala when my prepaid local phone rang. I answered, and a woman I did not know greeted me with an apology for having received my number from an unnamed mutual colleague. For a few moments, our conversation was general and flattering, with my caller saying how much she appreciated my work. She then began discussing the outcomes of a high-profile government program for "zero hunger," which involved a significant amount of money and political capital to eliminate Guatemala's pernicious challenge of childhood undernutrition and growth stunting.[39] I noticed that the voice on the other end echoed, as though my unidentified caller was in a tiled bathroom, and I started hearing papers shuffling. I realized I was talking to a whistleblower in the Ministry of Health. She was disturbed that the government was claiming success while evaluation data showed the programming was having little impact, and there were indications that funds had been misdirected.[40]

I quickly took down notes of statistics from program evaluation data that had been hidden. The whole call only lasted a few minutes. My caller encouraged me to "tell my friends" what she had shared and hung up. I always question my role as a foreign researcher and the value that I might be able to bring to efforts in Guatemala, as I work alongside brilliant and committed Guatemalan activists, scholars, and practitioners. This call made me realize that I could use the privilege of my foreignness to support the local leaders in their efforts for transparency and a health sector that works for the whole population. Word of the program failures and efforts to obscure them got out. People were angry—again—at the power structures that enable glossy billboards and catchy slogans but yield systematic change no deeper than the thickness of their paper and cheap rhymes. Endemic corruption plagues the Guatemalan government and health sector, with several scandals resulting in the resignation and prosecution of two recent presidents and a vice president.

Corruption and poor oversight were also key challenges that led to the downfall of the SIAS program for delivering primary care to communities. Government-contracted NGOs were responsible for hiring and supervising mobile health teams, but oversight of the mobile teams was erratic. NGO coordinators often only saw the mobile teams once a month and relied on the teams themselves to self-regulate their day-to-day activities. Mobile teams submitted patient health data in a standardized spreadsheet to the departmental Ministry of Health office, but they otherwise had only ad hoc contact with the government health infrastructure. The structure of the SIAS program was theoretically standardized across the country and gave the NGOs administering the program very little leeway to adapt program structures and systems to local needs.

Mobile team members were supposed to oversee and train the community health workers within their municipalities. However, I found a lackadaisical approach to their monitoring capacity. On one occasion, Delia, a mobile health nurse, told me that the CHWs are not really of any help to them. She cited the example of a community health worker whose village we had visited that day who could not explain to a new mother how to give the standard neonatal vitamins or what they were for. "That mother won't use those. She has no idea what she's doing, and the CHW can't really help her," Delia said. Indeed, there was an air of futility about many of the activities of the mobile teams and their work with the CHWs.

Chimaltenango was the birthplace of high-quality CHW programs for the country through an NGO called the Carroll Behrhorst Foundation, which meticulously trained CHWs in both preventive and curative health services.[41] While the SIAS program paid homage in some ways to these legacy programs, it could not maintain the same high standards of care when scaled at the national level and administered through a wide variety of NGOs. During a monthly CHW meeting in Acatenango, I was disappointed to find that the CHWs could not accurately tell me how to use ORT, one of the cornerstones of basic primary care in Guatemala. This was just one small example of how CHW training was not uniformly provided to enable delivery of safe and accurate health advice.

The true legacy of SIAS may be the blurring of public and private sectors within health-seeking, but lack of oversight, exacerbated by poor funding, was ultimately its demise. This led to huge regional disparities in access to and quality of primary care, depending on the contracted NGO and their staff. Some did incredible jobs, providing care in first languages and building deep relationships within communities. Others—too many others—were taking the lucrative government contracts and providing substandard services. The system had too few redundancies in fiduciary supervision, leading to high levels of corruption and seepage of government funds into pockets that never intended to improve the health of the rural poor. Similarly, both during and after the fall of the SIAS program, health posts are vulnerable to corruption because of the low wages and weak supervision of staff. The government system experiences frequent stockouts of the basic medicines that health posts are meant have, leading to opportunities for price gouging and for-profit sales.

Conclusion

Without question, the living memory of genocide and the ongoing trauma of peacetime violence affect the health of Maya communities. They embody the effects of physical and structural violence, the forces of which continue to create barriers to health care. The violent othering of Maya peoples that began at conquest was of embodied selves. The Maya were subjugated into colonial political and economic structures, but they were also colonized by binary ideologies that continue to marginalize them—Maya/ladino, clean/ dirty, developed/backward. Colonizing cognitive structures position Maya thought and lifeways at the margins of Guatemalan society, and through othering, the Indigenous is remade as foreign.[42]

False binaries play into the hands of neoliberal metrics by eliding what really happens. For example, low Maya use rates of the government health system are used as a rationale for limiting the expansion of services, justifying exclusion as evidence-based practice and neoliberal economic common sense. Ministry of Health and other government officials can say the numbers do not add up for further expenditures within Maya communities. They can conclude that Maya communities do not want government health care. Binaries allow metrics and the decisions ostensibly based on them to homogenize diverse groups, where "the Maya" can be reduced to a single racist trope and dismissed. Numbers should not be allowed to "speak for themselves" in global health. Health system metrics can become tools of abandonment, corruption, and unjust power structures.[43]

Power is exerted across the metasystems of neoliberalism and global health and throughout the hierarchies they maintain. If the labor of bodies is controlled as a means of production, then systems of manipulation and tacit control create what Michel Foucault deems "docile bodies."[44] Health systems (and access to them) are a locus of control of bodies and, by extension, of populations.[45] Yet, just as conquistadores underestimated the resolve of the Maya population to resist ethnocide, Foucault fails to fully explain or locate resistance to dominant systems of bodily control. If, in fact, the collective control and regulation of the bodies of contemporary populations is largely due to the systematic medicalization of society, what of the agency of those marginalized from health systems?[46]

In the recent past, the internal armed conflict was fought to control Mayan bodies, to dictate where they could be and what they could have in Guatemalan society. In the present, structures of care and provider interactions show Maya communities that the human right to health is not really meant for them. But they are more than docile bodies, however much Guatemalan health system structures and global health programs might want to imagine otherwise. They choose when and how to interact with a health system not designed for them, reinforcing their right to this choice, even if it means forgoing government health services. The reality of inaccessible government health services further opens up the possibilities and allure of the private-sector health care marketplace. As we will see in chapter 4, many rural Maya care-seekers understand that quality of care and cost are conflated, and they seek health care outside the government system. The power to choose feels like freedom, but it is an illusory trick of neoliberalism.

4 Turning Diarrhea into Dinero: Market-Driven Health Services

When our children get really sick, we take them to the doctor if we have money. But, if not, we just wait for God's decision.
—mother and focus-group participant, village of Acatenango

In our village, we do not have a doctor, and the children need one. They suffer because it is difficult for us to take them to town to see a doctor.
—mother in Panaj

I first met Felix at the Pollo Campero fast-food restaurant on the edge of the central park in Chimaltenango. I had been referred to him by the Guatemala City–based national offices of Omnilife, a multilevel marketing company focused on nutritional supplements and natural remedies, as the leading seller and most knowledgeable sales representative in Chimaltenango. That afternoon, Felix and a business partner were the picture of upwardly mobile ambition: dressed in knit polo shirts and carrying their attaché bags, they looked ready to give a sales pitch to a new client. They seemed excited and a little nervous to have the chance to talk about Omnilife to a foreigner. Although I had explained over the telephone and again when we met in person that I was a researcher interested in Omnilife and not a prospective vendor, I could not sway Felix from his recruitment sales pitch that afternoon. As we ate our chicken, Felix extolled the virtues of the company.

Felix said that he used to live in a dirt-floored, badly built house in his hometown and always had to worry about putting the next meal on the table. Felix reported that, since he began working as an Omnilife vendor four years earlier, his standard of living had vastly improved. He bought a used car, traveled to Omnilife conventions at resorts in Central America and the Caribbean as rewards for high sales, and even built a new two-story "mansion." He told me, "Working in the fields is hard. Omnilife has made my life so much better. My grandparents are poor, my parents are poor, but I am not poor. I think everyone should do it—there's no reason to be poor." Felix said he made about US$20,000 per year from his own product sales and an additional US$4,000 in annual bonuses for his recruits and their product sales, which he proudly reminded me was a very high wage for Guatemala. In this respect, Felix differs from other Omnilife vendors, who typically sell a far lesser volume of products and earn far less.

During my initial meeting with Felix and at all subsequent Omnilife vendor events I attended, the products themselves took a distinct back-seat to discussing the lifestyle aspects of the company. Felix brought some samples of the products for me to try. He insisted that he could taste the difference between an Omnilife "extra pure" bottle of water that sells for double the cost of the regular bottled water we had ordered from the res-taurant, and he was a little disappointed that I could not make the same fine distinction. Many of Omnilife's products are vitamin powders that you mix with water. Felix told me that one of these powders had cured his wife's painful ovarian cysts and kept her from dying. Omnilife bills its products as healthy and all natural, although many products contain either sucrose or fructose as their first ingredient and have a fairly extensive list of additional chemical ingredients.

Vendors know little about the products they sell, and the indications for the individual products are vague. Felix told me that everyone must choose the right products for them, adding that you could mix several different powders in one drink and "nothing [bad] would happen." When I asked how mixing different products would affect their efficacy, he said that more is always better, and you would see results more quickly the more Omnil-ife products you took. Obviously, this "more is better" is an effective sales strategy, as Felix's customers could only benefit more by purchasing greater quantities of products, but the actual efficacy of the individual products themselves seems questionable. However, while Felix is very focused on making sales, I never felt that he was operating from a position of deception: he truly believes in the life-changing power of Omnilife and its products.

This chapter widens the lens to include oral rehydration therapy (ORT) in market-driven health care venues within the interstitial spaces that shifting health and development programs create for the growth of private-sector health services and commodities, which further introduce opportunities and burdens of choice. Felix was the shining exception to the norm of how market-driven health goods and services impact the rural poor. More typically, the poor are doubly affected by quasi-pharmaceutical pyramid schemes that both recruit them as low-level vendors with promises of huge profits and by misinforming them as consumers as to the efficacy and benefits of the products. Social obligations and aspirations encourage the purchase of expensive "miracle" products whose shifting indications always match customers' symptoms.

In this chapter, I investigate the consequences of untrained vendors dispensing health advice along with dubious products to the parents of children with diarrhea. I explore individuals' choices, bodily autonomy, and power in health-seeking by prioritizing costly private-sector services. High prestige products and services reinforce the notion that health equals wealth but too often yield empty promises of the high quality of care for which they are an illusory proxy. I also describe traditional healers as a culturally and financially accessible option within Maya communities and the role they play in contemporary fee-for-service treatment-seeking. Finally, I discuss how short-term medical missions and the philanthropic sector contribute to the pluralistic health care landscape. By examining these elements of market-driven health care, we gain further perspective on the widely held belief in Chimaltenango that health requires purchasing power. The neoliberal economy creates a desire for a freedom of choice within a health care marketplace, but true choices remain out of reach for many in Guatemala.

The (Neo)colonial Birth of Neoliberalism in Latin America

The current pluralistic health care landscape in Guatemala has been forged by the neoliberal economy and its principals of privatization and profit optimization. A long history of colonial extraction shaped the current Guatemalan neoliberal economy, and a possibly gentler but nonetheless pernicious extraction continues through contemporary foreign aid structures and trade agreements. Here I explore the rise of neoliberalism in Latin America to trace the emergence of foreign aid and global health structures.

Mercantilism in sixteenth-century Spanish-occupied America sought to increase the power and wealth of Spain to disadvantage colonial rivals England and Portugal. Spanish conquistadors defeated Maya groups in what is now Guatemala. Many explanations of their seemingly easy success have been proposed, from the advantages of guns over spears to the lack of unification of the empires, but the greatest ally of the Spanish was infectious disease.[1] Smallpox alone is thought to have killed between one-third to one-half of the populations of the Aztec and Incan empires. The accumulation of power was measured in bullion, both gold and silver. The mercantilist policy was to ensure that exports exceeded imports, allowing for increases in stored wealth for Spain. The first mechanism for achieving this was extensive mining in the "New World," and the second was retaining control over commerce in the colonies in order to have the upper hand in trade. The mercantilist system remained intact for nearly 300 years.[2]

The labor of Indigenous people generated the wealth of the colonial Spanish economy. Indigenous people labored in mines and in fields to produce wealth for the Crown. Some political historians have even proposed that the weakening of the mercantilist system did not occur until the Indigenous population experienced sharp decline due to conquest and disease.[3] Spain and other colonial powers used Latin American territories as sources of precious metals and other natural resources, viewing the labor potential of the remaining Indigenous populations as just another resource to be controlled.[4]

By the 1820s, most of Spanish-colonized America had gained political independence, and the next half-century was marked by withdrawal from the world economy. Guatemala achieved independence in 1821.[5] Independence was in name only for Indigenous populations; the emerging class of Creole (people of European descent born in Latin America) landowners became the new controllers of land, labor, and wealth. With the Industrial Revolution of the nineteenth century, Latin America again became important to the global capitalist economy as a source of raw materials and as a market for manufactured goods.[6] Creole landowners managed plantations of sugar and, later, oil and rubber production. The plantations used the labor of Indigenous workers and made only marginal profits that were spent on manufactured imports. Hence, the labor of the Indigenous peons, not unlike enslaved people in the Caribbean at that time, fueled the industrialization of Europe and the United States.[7]

Since the 1980s, economic policy in Latin America and globally, has emphasized neoliberalism, based on the principle that market forces and competition provide the most efficient means of distribution of capital in society.[8] This approach has exacerbated existing inequalities, both between high-income and global majority countries and socioeconomic differences within countries. In considering the rise of global capitalism in Latin America, Brazilian economist Theotônio Dos Santos presciently stated at the advent of neoliberalism: "In a world market of commodities, capital, and even of labor power, we see that the relations produced by this market are unequal and combined—unequal because development of parts of the system occurs at the expense of other parts."[9]

Countries classed as low- and middle-income by the World Bank continue to be dependent on imports, minimizing the potential for accrual of capital within the economy. Structural adjustment of development loans in the 1970s was widespread in the Latin America as prior development loans came due, through which the International Monetary Fund (IMF) and World Bank compelled privatization and foreign investment to refinance. Latin American economies became locked into an endless aid-debt cycle that drains profits in the form of debt payments and foreign investment.[10] In *Open Veins of Latin America*, Eduardo Galeano railed against this form of aid: "The IMF was created to institutionalize Wall Street's financial dominion over the whole planet, when the dollar first achieved hegemony as international currency after World War II. It has never been untrue to its master."[11] Social economist Andre Gunder Frank further contended that Latin America must break ties with global capitalist structures to end the exploitive relationships that keep the region underdeveloped.[12] As prescient as they were, these warnings now seem almost quaint in an increasingly privatized and market-driven neoliberal economy. Certainly, since the 1970s, economic development indicators for the Latin American region as a whole and for Guatemala have improved, but the benefits have not been shared equally within societies.

In particular, economic development efforts in Latin America have not improved the lives of Indigenous peoples on a widespread scale. As Norbert Lechner argued, "Globalization aggravates the social distances internal to each society. This effect is especially troublesome in Latin America, which is marked already by some of the highest inequalities in the world."[13] Economic reforms have left most Latin American countries with neoliberal states that prioritize private and market-driven solutions to distribute public goods, such as health care and education.[14] Despite being Central America's largest economy and boasting stable economic growth across three decades, Guatemala still has among the highest levels of income inequality in the region.[15] Guatemala's status as an upper-middle-income country belies the very low federal taxation rates, resulting in low funding for social goods like health care and public health infrastructure. This low tax base, largely due to tax evasion and weak governance, underlies persistent lags in development measures and inequality.[16]

In Latin America, severe rural-urban disparities persist, with poverty most concentrated in rural areas.[17] Within national economies throughout Latin America, rural areas become satellites of urban areas, just as the countries of the region are dependent on global economic powerhouses. Although Guatemala has experienced urbanization common throughout the region in the past three decades, 48 percent of the population continue to live in rural areas.[18] Since rural populations in Guatemala are more often Indigenous Maya, they are geographically and structurally further from the benefits of urban economic growth.

Impacts of the Contemporary Guatemalan Economy on Health

The Guatemalan economy has followed the broad trends of economic usurpation under Spanish colonialism and weak development and interaction in the world market since independence. It has been shaped by, the neocolonialism of US industries, such as the infamous United Fruit Company. Guatemala's per capita gross domestic income was $4,317 in 2020; yet income disparities skew this average. The richest 10 percent of households received 51 percent of the nation's gross total income and the poorest 50 percent of households only 12 percent.[19] Inflation has recently exceeded annual growth of the gross domestic product (GDP).[20] Further, Guatemala has gotten locked into a foreign aid-debt cycle, with current debt servicing totaling approximately 7 percent of all exports of goods and services. Guatemala's urban population now comprises about 52 percent of the nation's 17 million total population, meaning that rapidly growing urban areas have received more attention, development, and infrastructure at the expense of rural development.[21] Current World Bank estimates show that 50 percent of the Guatemalan population live in poverty and 29 percent in extreme poverty.[22]

Guatemala's top three official exports are coffee, sugar, and bananas, but the probable top three foreign-currency earners are foreign remittances, tourism, and drug trafficking.[23] Further, forces of globalization and the export of agricultural products to high-income countries exacerbate existing power inequalities in the agricultural sector. New cash crops, or nontraditional crops grown exclusively for export like broccoli and rasp-berries, are sought-after exports, but inexperience in growing these crops and price fluctuations make them a serious financial gamble for small-scale farmers. Cash crops require expensive inputs of pesticides and seed, and farm-to-market systems where farmers must sell to intermediary brokers cut into the profits of individual farmers. The failure of small-scale farmers further consolidates land and money in the hands of the wealthy when they default on loans for agricultural inputs and are forced to sell.[24] Guate-mala has garment factories and other light industry, although a majority of manufacturing facilities are foreign-owned, often facilitated through trade agreements. Land-lease programs for factory complexes have been a corner-stone of a trade agreement with South Korea, among others. South Korea has, in turn, undertaken some development projects, including donation of the maternity ward at the Chimaltenango government hospital.

Privatization and Fee-for-Service Health Facilities

The shift toward privatization of health care in Guatemala mirrors trends in global health and the global neoliberal economy as a whole. Although medical providers have long had private practices in Guatemala's urban centers, health system privatization in Guatemala began in earnest with the vanguard of philanthropic health and international development organizations starting in the 1950s. For example, the Behrhorst Clinic and Hospital, founded in 1962 by Kansas-born Dr. Carroll Behrhorst, pioneered the nonprofit private health care sector.[25] Behrhorst first came to Guate-mala as part of a medical mission in the late 1950s. With support from the Lutheran Church, Behrhorst aimed to bring health care to a Kaqchikel Maya population of 140,000 in the Chimaltenango area who had no access to health services.[26] Behrhorst knew that he could not provide adequate numbers of physicians to care for the population, but he believed that local community members could be trained to diagnose and treat many com-mon illnesses. He designed a system in which doctors trained local health promoters. Costs were kept low in the hospital, as family members prepared food and provided basic nursing care for the patients.[27] The organization's spirit reflected a "health for the people, by the people" ideal. Further rec-ognizing that curative medicine alone could not address the poor health status of the Kaqchikel population of Chimaltenango, Behrhorst and his colleagues began programs to address issues of malnutrition, land tenure, agricultural production, and population control.[28]

In 1975, the WHO cited the Behrhorst program as a model for effective health promotion in underresourced regions.[29] The global health of the time emphasized primary care and decentralized health system delivery models. Following the 1976 earthquake, a Guatemalan government health official stated that the Behrhorst Clinic had the best organized health service in the country. The extreme violence of the early 1980s impeded but did not extinguish the Behrhorst health initiatives: by the end of 1983, only eighteen of forty-five trained health promoters had survived.[30] Apart from a brief period during the violence of the early 1980s, Behrhorst continued his work in Chimaltenango until his death in 1990. He was a widely recognized and beloved figure in the department, having garnered the trust and respect of the Kaqchikel people over his many years of work with them as a colleague rather than a savior.[31]

The pressures of the neoliberal economy have meant that the Behrhorst Clinic now operates on a fee-for-service basis commensurate with pricing at other private clinics in Chimaltenango; a basic consultation costs 30 Q (Guatemalan quetzales or US$4.29). Three or four doctors are on duty each weekday, and they rotate responsibilities for covering the evening and overnight shifts. The Behrhorst Clinic offers a full range of specialty services, including dermatology and gynecology through regular visits from specialists one day a week. However, patient numbers have dwindled in recent years. Older staff members remember when they had to work steadily all day to get through all of the patients, whereas now the long benches lining the breezeways around the hospital facility are often emptied of the day's patients by 10 a.m. The inpatient hospital rooms are almost always completely empty, bereft of the bustling of Indigenous patients and their caretaking family members of earlier times.[32] Poor Maya patients can no longer afford the Behrhorst Clinic for surgical procedures, apart from when a foreign medical team comes for a week of volunteer service. Further, the staff of the Behrhorst Clinic are no longer majority Maya. Instead, nearly all of the doctors, nurses, and even support staff are mostly ladino.[33]

Much of the community programming described during the halcyon days of Dr. Behrhorst's time at the clinic no longer exists.[34] However, the philanthropic and community-engaged work of Behrhorst continues through a non-governmental organization (NGO) that now operates as a separate entity from the hospital. After a decade of institutional disentanglement, the spin-off NGO's primarily Kaqchikel Maya staff provides essential community initiatives, such as clean water systems and nutrition education through community gardens. The NGO's funding comes from foreign grants and donations.

With funding from the government, the Behrhorst Clinic oversaw ambulatory teams of doctors and nurses in four municipalities of Chimaltenango for more than a decade through the Guatemalan government's extension of coverage program (PEC for its Spanish acronym) until the program's end in 2014. These teams, in turn, trained local community health workers. As described in chapter 3, the government's PEC program was designed to fulfill the government promise of health care for everyone. Mirroring a global trend in neoliberal health delivery, the government outsourced the lowest tier of primary care services to NGOs, which coordinated the mobile health teams to visit each village within their catchment area at least once monthly. The NGO teams administered government-funded programs such as routine vaccination and nutritional supplements for young children.

The idea behind PEC was that the NGOs already had relationships with communities and would be better able to provide accessible care. However, the reality was messier—some NGOs worked to fulfill their mandates while others took the money and delivered little care. In 2013, a government audit found high levels of corruption within the PEC program, and the program was discontinued in 2014 without a clear substitute in place. Further, rigidity in PEC program structures meant that NGOs, like Behrhorst Clinic, were given little flexibility to adapt programs to community contexts, despite this being a goal of the program.[35] The outsourcing model did not work for effective national primary care coverage. Unfortunately, the model Dr. Behrhorst developed to use the hospital facility as a place to teach community health workers through intensive classes and hands-on clinical experience had to be abandoned at the end of PEC out of economic necessity.

To address competition from other private health facilities, the Behrhorst Clinic capitalizes on its previous reputation as the highest-quality health care in the department. The hospital administration implemented a billboard and radio ad campaign, complete with jingle, "Come to the hospital of the *gringo*. It's the best!" The clinic's reputation of high-quality care and deep history of serving Maya communities still draws paying customers. Prices are the same at the Behrhorst for everyone, and those who cannot pay are referred to the government hospital. Payments for all procedures must be made upfront, even in an emergency situation that I observed involving a woman who had been cut across the face with a machete.

While the vibrancy and patient volume of the Behrhorst Clinic has declined with the cessation of external funding, it continues to provide essential health care to those who can pay. Children who present with diarrhea are typically triaged using the government guidelines (the Plan A, B, C triage algorithm) and then sent to the in-house laboratory for a fecal test to check for high bacterial and parasitic loads. Accordingly, Behrhorst clinicians do not recommend or prescribe antibiotics or antiparasitic medications without a clear diagnosis of a diarrheal pathogen. Behrhorst doctors largely adhere to their policy of promoting ORT as a safe and less costly and invasive treatment in comparison to treating children for dehydration with intravenous (IV) fluids. One doctor told me, "We have to argue with mothers sometimes. They bring their children all the way here, and they want an IV. They don't always want just a drink from the pharmacy, so we have to explain it to them." That said, either pressure from paying patients or delayed treatment-seeking resulting in a more severe condition means that some children receive IV therapy to treat their diarrhea.

The Behrhorst Clinic is one of many private fee-for-service clinics operating in Chimaltenango, and their services are too expensive to be accessible for all. In the eyes of many rural Maya, health and the ability to seek health care are the exclusive domain of the wealthy. Amid the nods and words of agreement of her neighbors, one focus-group participant in Panaj matter-of-factly explained, "We are poor and cannot take our children to the doctor often. We do not take our children to the doctor until they are seriously ill—unlike rich people, who take their children to the doctor to be examined even if they are not sick. Imagine, even if they are not sick!" Indeed, as we talked in the small dirt yard of one of the women, looking down toward the crossroads of the village, the idea of taking all sick kids to a health care provider, let alone the healthy ones, seemed like pure fantasy. The transition of health care from public good to marketplace commodity positions patients as consumers who are financially and even morally responsible for their own care.[36] It facilitates further government abandonment of responsibility for the human right to health.

Pharmacies and the Commodification of Health

Further populating the complex neoliberal health care landscape, pharmacies are a critical source of treatment for childhood sickness, including diarrhea. The term "pharmacy" spans a wide gamut of establishments and vendors, including government pharmacies, private pharmacies, and individual vendors who sell pharmaceuticals in shops and market stands. In my research, pharmacies were widely reported to be good sources of ORT by both Maya and ladino participants.[37] Another study of treatment-seeking for children in Guatemala found that 30 percent of children who were treated for diarrhea were seen by a pharmacist, which is unsurprising since childhood diarrhea is so common.[38] Generally speaking, people in the Chimaltenango Department have a high opinion of biomedical pharmaceuticals, and many believe that they are the best possible recourse during a bout of sickness. The convenience of being able to pick up basic medicines along with other household goods at a local shop is an important factor in treatment-seeking decisions.

In 1997, the government opened a network of pharmacies as part of the Drug Access Program (PROAM). The aim of the program is to make pharmaceuticals accessible and affordable to everyone in Guatemala, and it includes pharmacies at the departmental and municipal levels as well as the stocks of drugs used by health centers, health posts, and community health workers. The government negotiates group contract pricing for the basic drug list available within the PROAM network.[39] Their pricing for powder sachets and bottled solution of oral rehydration salts (ORS) is competitive, when they have them in stock, but not considerably lower than private pharmacies.

Similar to PROAM pharmacies, the staff in private pharmacies uniformly suggested antibiotics or antiparasitic medications when I inquired about what treatment they would recommend for a hypothetical eighteen-month-old with diarrhea. At only one (private) pharmacy did the salesperson recommend that ORT be used in conjunction with the medication suggested. Particularly in the private pharmacy context, these recommendations are perhaps to be expected since antibiotics and antiparasitics are far more expensive than ORS packets, which cost only a few quetzales (about US$0.20). At several of the pharmacies, ORT packets and bottled solution were available when requested, but the stock was faded and dusty, underscoring the fact that ORT sales are not an emphasis for pharmacy staff.

The Behrhorst Clinic operates its own twenty-four-hour pharmacy at the front of the hospital building in Chimaltenango. Their pharmacy manager and other staff had little to no training in pharmaceuticals, which is usually the case even for staff in the most polished-looking private pharmacies. The Behrhorst pharmacy fills prescriptions written by its clinic doctors as well as sells medicines directly to customers on the street. The pharmacy has a wide variety of competitively priced bottled and powdered ORS solutions, and it sells approximately 300 bottles and 50 packets of ORS each month, again indicating the marked preference for the bottled solutions. Unlike most pharmacies, Behrhorst pharmacy instructs its staff to provide directions to parents purchasing ORT on how to administer the solution appropriately; however, in my observation, this step was typically rushed or forgotten.

Since regulation of pharmaceutical sales is weak, vendors of an ever-changing variety of pharmaceuticals abound in local markets. Laid out on blankets and tables among vegetables, laundry detergent, and hair gel, medications, most often antibiotics, are a typical and expected part of the marketplace landscape (figure 4.1). While these market vendors have no formal knowledge of pharmaceuticals other than anecdotal evidence gleaned from personal experience, they always have something on hand to recommend for whatever condition you might be looking to treat. Purchasers of biomedical medicines in the marketplace are both reliant on the vendors for advice and willing to believe that the quantity of medicine they are able to purchase will be sufficient to restore health.[40] In a system where medications are not controlled, issues of antibiotic misuse and resistance become very serious.

An additional part of the market-driven pharmaceutical scene are the many market vendors and shops selling "natural" remedies. Sellers of these products told me that their most popular remedies are for gastrointestinal health and male sexual "vitality." Pricing for these products vary: some are cheaper than biomedical pharmaceuticals and others cost more. However, I have not found that these "natural" stores formed an important source of treatment for children. There seems to be a surge in demand by urban ladinos and foreigners for natural medicines that draw on spiritualist beliefs that are not a part of traditional Maya healing.

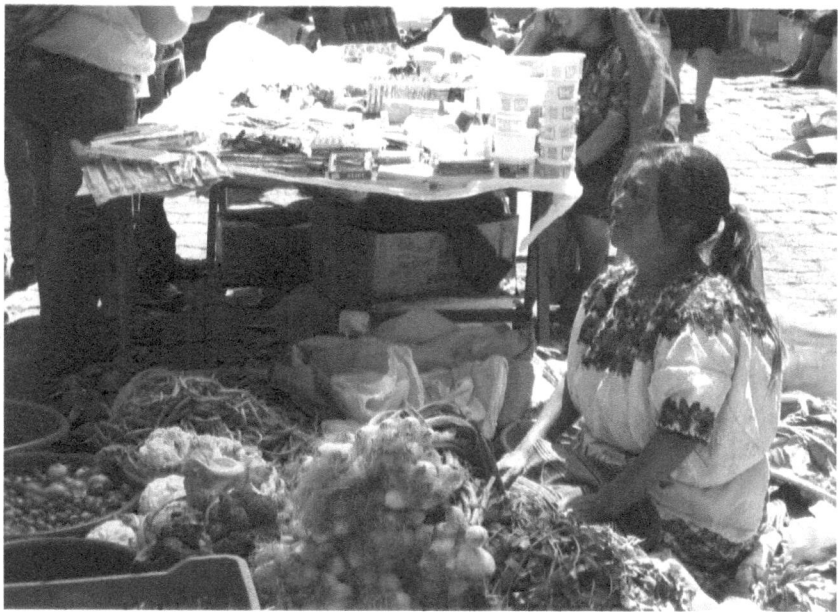

Figure 4.1
Marketplace pharmaceuticals in Acatenango.

The Omnipresence of Omnilife and the Multilevel Marketing of Wellness

Omnilife is a multinational corporation that sells vitamins and other health supplements and remedies, including products claiming to be useful for ORT. As we saw in Felix's example at the start of the chapter, Omnilife follows a direct sales model by selling its products through licensed vendors who earn money by selling the products at a set rate of profit markup and by recruiting other vendors. Founded in Mexico in 1991, the majority of Omnilife's distribution centers and vendors continue to be in Central America; however, Omnilife is a registered company in nineteen countries worldwide, including the United States, Russia, and India. Omnilife has a strong presence in Guatemala: it has now been operating in the country for thirteen years and grosses approximately US$12 million annually.[41] Direct sales and multilevel marketing have become popular strategies in low- and middle-income countries with the rise of Omnilife and other multinationals such as Amway.[42] The aspirational message of high potential earnings for vendors with few economic opportunities as well as a consumer base desirous of "strong" packaged remedies makes Guatemala a location ripe for Omnilife's multilevel marketing and direct sales strategies.[43] The packaged nature of Omnilife's health supplement quasi-pharmaceutical products makes them appealing in the same way as, and in some cases indistinguishable from, pharmaceuticals.

Multilevel marketing strategies rely on large numbers of small-scale investors and on the continuous recruitment of new investors and customers to fund payments to existing investors; across multilevel marketing strategies, 90 percent of investors do not have their expectations for returns on investment met.[44] After attending a few of the sporadic meetings of Omnilife vendors in Chimaltenango, Felix invited me to accompany him to a "top vendors" meeting in Guatemala City, where, he said, the vendors learned about the properties of and uses for the products. I had to become an authorized vendor in order to attend the meeting, so I became one of Felix's recruits and paid the 170 Q(US$25) initiation fee. Though a great disappointment to Felix, whose visions of profit shares from a US recruit loomed large, I never ordered or sold any Omnilife products. This, I thought, was my chance—I would be able to learn about exactly what the products are good for and how some of them are conceptualized as ORT. Maybe it made sense that the local Chimaltenango meetings were all about sales, but this would be where the actual product education took place!

In a meeting hall of a midrange hotel in Guatemala City, the vendors gathered for their midafternoon meeting. The crowd of about 200 vendors was a mix of largely Indigenous men and some Indigenous women. Loud music blared through oversized speakers, and Omnilife beverages were sold at the door, where an entry fee of US$2 was charged. Amid much fanfare, the meeting's leader ran to the front of the room and began an impassioned testimonial about the many ways that Omnilife has improved his life. Attendees clapped and shouted words of affirmation. Indeed, Omnilife draws on charismatic leadership and faith-based models of group-building, such as call and response activities.[45] As the afternoon wore on, we heard testimonials from other vendors and repeated explanations of how the Omnilife vendor system operates. Depending on your volume of sales, you can buy the products at increasingly reduced wholesale prices for a larger profit margin; you cannot sell products from a store; and you receive a bonus plus profit shares from the sales of three generations of your recruits. A marker board was used to carefully explain this process and to draw out the pyramid structure of profits, dispelling any doubt that it is indeed a pyramid scheme.

Throughout the afternoon, I wondered if the vendor-attendees would not already be very well aware of the information being presented, yet the responsive crowd was far from bored. Toward the end of the three-hour meeting, there was a "product education" segment during which vendors were reminded to push sales of two different products: one powdered vitamin supplement for "vitality" and a liquid syrup for "digestive health." Nothing more specific than these vague uses were given; discussion centered on how "good" the products were and the possibilities for profit margins. Essentially, the meeting served as something of a pep rally for the vendors, reigniting their interest in and commitment to the Omnilife way of life rather than providing them with product knowledge that would help them select the best products for any given condition that a customer might have. On the drive back to Chimaltenango, Felix talked animatedly about the meeting and about his future plans for increased sales. He said he planned to buy a trunkload of products and drive them out to the rural markets on a more regular basis. He has had some success with this sales strategy in the past. "The rural people," he said, "are hungry for health. They will buy these products that they need."

When I pressed Felix and other Omnilife vendors on how they decided which products to recommend for patients with particular conditions, they said they relied on firsthand knowledge of and experience with the products themselves. Felix said he also reads Omnilife publications, including the company magazine, to learn more about the products, though my own perusal of these publications again revealed an emphasis on testimonials and sales techniques. However, Felix and other Omnilife vendors repeatedly reiterated to me that Omnilife is exceedingly equal opportunity in that you do not have to be able to read or even speak Spanish well to be a good vendor. This means that the written promotional and educational materials would not be accessible to all vendors, let alone their largely rural Indigenous customers. Further, the vast majority of vendors and clients alike do not have the social position, training, and experience to be critical of the promises of a multinational corporation like Omnilife and its methods of operation. As I talked with more vendors and customers, it became increasingly clear to me that careful education in the appropriate use of the products is not a priority of Omnilife.

My specific interest in understanding Omnilife's promotional and sales processes was focused on the use of some of the products as ORS solutions. Although vendors all agreed that their products made more effective ORS solutions for children than the free or low-cost packets given out at health posts, they invariably recommended a different selection of products for this purpose. Felix was opinionated on the topic, saying that rural parents did not know any better and gave their children unhealthy drinks like Coca-Colas when they have diarrhea, and he urged that they should be using healthier solutions, like any of the wide variety of drinks and powders offered by Omnilife. When I pointed out that some form of sugar was the first ingredient in several of these products, Felix became extremely defensive, saying that the benefits of the vitamin content were what sets Omnilife apart from all other ORS solutions. It also became clear that he did not realize that ingredients like sucrose and fructose are chemical names for sugar.

Of course, the cost of Omnilife products that would be used for ORT purposes is far more than the cost of government packets or even other commercial products available at pharmacies. Depending on the specific product recommended, Omnilife "digestive" remedies used for ORT can range in price from 3 Q (US$0.43) per packet to 12 Q (US$1.70) for a bottle of vitamin water to as high as 72 Q (US$10) for a bottle of syrup. In comparison to even the private pharmacy pricing discussed in the previous section, Omnilife prices are significantly higher. A sort of attainable (or at least conceivably attainable) elitism seems to be the modus operandi of many Omnilife vendors with whom I spoke and who sell products in rural areas. As one vendor in Comalapa put it, "The thing about Omnilife products is that everyone wants them because not everyone can get them." An upwardly mobile Indigenous man himself, he added, "The peasants come into town each week to the market, and they see and hear how good our products are. These people are poor and often can't afford them [Omnilife products] right away, but it makes them want to afford them." As in the case of access to private health facilities, the concept that health is for those who can pay is reinforced. Even the most marginalized in society, those who should be able to rely on public goods like health care, are shown that health is something to be paid for like any other market good.

By creating social cachet surrounding the purchase of Omnilife brand products used as ORT, Omnilife vendors hope to create a market where people forgo cheaper products in favor of their own, supposedly superior product. Vendors are often friends and family or at least a fellow Indigenous neighbor with whom rural customers can identify. Omnilife sales rely on the trust relationships present in rural communities to sell products and to make people believe that no other brand is worth purchasing. It is socially desirable to be seen with Omnilife products touted as ORS, even if you cannot afford enough to give your sick child a dosage that would be effective. I have seen unopened or slightly used bottles of Omnilife products sitting in windowsills and on shelves in many low-income households, suggesting that the products are being hoarded for later use because of their cost or simply kept as status symbols.[46] The social cachet of using expensive packaged treatments comes at the cost of actually treating childhood diarrhea.

Omnilife encourages its vendors to think of selling their health products as a public service. It is unsurprising, then, when seepage between the public and private sector occurs, particularly when low-paid community health workers (CHWs) supplement their income by becoming quasi-pharmaceutical vendors. At the health post closest to the village of Panaj, Carlos, the CHW in Simajuleu, was lax about the hours that he opened the health post. The women in the village frequently shared their frustration about having made the long walk to the post only to find it closed, as in Rosario's experience of seeking care for baby Efraín in the introduction. After a couple of attempted visits, I finally found Carlos in the health post one afternoon. I was asking him my usual questions about what kinds of problems he sees most frequently and which medications he is able to offer when I noticed two shelves of Omnilife products. I started asking questions about the Omnilife products, and Carlos said he had them in the post as a service to the customers and that many of them preferred them to the government products. He said that for a child with diarrhea, he will recommend one of the Omnilife bottles of vitamin water, but that if a mother cannot pay for it, he will sell her a government ORS packet if he has any left.

Although CHWs are intended to be volunteers for their communities who are only compensated for the time they spend away from other income-generating activities, Carlos in Simajuleu has found a way to make more money operating the health post. There is little time and money for oversight of the CHWs, so it is unsurprising that some promoters chose to add other money-making ventures onto their official health post activities. I only saw Omnilife products in one other health post in the Comalapa municipality, though most of my visits were with announced trips of the mobile health teams. While Omnilife rules prohibit sales from a store, they do not explicitly ban sales from health posts, which are technically not run as for-profit businesses. As a result, there is a gray area for community CHWs to take advantage of their position and earn extra money as vendors of Omnilife. CHW encouragement of Omnilife purchases rather than the medicines available at low cost through the government service makes them seem of superior quality, bolstering attitudes that better health can be purchased with a greater expenditure of money.

The distinctive Omnilife branding on products is widely recognized, and people's trust in their effectiveness is strengthened by the social networks through which they are sold.[47] This kind of trust is hard to come by in encounters with in the government health system for Maya communities. Rather than being put off by the high cost of Omnilife products, potential customers trust and aspire to purchase them *because* of the high cost.[48] In this regard, Omnilife reflects a widespread trend toward a growing preference for more expensive products purchased out-of-pocket in the private pharmaceutical sector instead of therapeutically similar low-cost products.[49] Public-sector products are seen as representing an inferior level of care and, as such, are sometimes rejected by the populations for whom they are intended.

The popularity of Omnilife demonstrates a desire for economic participation that seems to sidestep the inequities of entrenched macroeconomic and class structures. Vendors connect Omnilife to a specific vision of modernity, viewing affiliation with the company as a sign not just of economic gain but of status as a participant in a globalized neoliberal economy.[50] A desire to participate in the global economy has been an important shift within Maya communities in the postwar era, particularly through engaging in factory labor and cash cropping.[51] But the gains made by participation in the neoliberal economy are unequally distributed, of course, and not everyone can access Omnilife as a vendor or purchaser.[52] While the Omnilife strategy benefits some individuals, as we saw with Felix's experience, it can amplify existing inequalities within communities as well as within the global economy. The apex of the multinational Omnilife pyramid was built to enrich a global economic elite, not to rebuild the wealth of the Maya, whose pyramids lie in ruins.

Local Healers in the Pluralistic Care Landscape

In addition to private clinics and pharmaceutical vendors of various kinds, local healers are another key group embedded within community structures that influence mothers' decisions about treatment-seeking for diarrhea in their children and ORT usage. Local healers offer another private-sector option in the pluralistic health care landscape that is often more geographically and financially accessible than other options. Many local healers charge very modest fees for their services and will accept food and other in-kind goods as payment. However, local healers should not be positioned as in conflict with biomedical care; they are often a first stop for advice or are consulted alongside biomedical care. Even in the early 1970s, Kris Heggenhougen found that there were few practicing shamans or *curanderas* (traditional healers typically using plant remedies) in the Chimaltenango Department.[53] However, most villages do still have a local individual, typically an older woman, who is seen as knowledgeable about plant and home remedies and skilled in healing common ailments.

Given the challenges in accessing care through the government health system, health-seeking options outside of that system and embedded within communities are a vital point-of-entry to care. In contemporary practice, local healers provide treatments but also help navigate other health care options. As fellow community members, local healers often have a shared view of the distance, cost, potential for discrimination or mistreatment, and perceived quality of other sources of health care, and they can help guide health-seekers through the complex calculus of decision-making across these factors for their specific health condition and situation. Particularly for Indigenous women who have less mobility and access to resources in Guatemalan society, these trusted sources of local care and advice are central in shaping hierarchies of resort—when to seek what treatment and where— and supporting decisions based on them. Local "traditional" healers therefore have become de facto guides in traversing the contemporary neoliberal health care landscape and variable accessibility of its offerings.[54] Generally, the more rural a community is, the more likely community members are to know a local healer.[55]

Doña Merilda, my neighbor in Comalapa whom we met in chapter 1, is a Kaqchikel Maya healer who held consultations for patients in her house. Doña Merilda's mother was a renowned healer in Comalapa in her day, and her daughters have learned the remedies as well, although they do not yet practice as healers. Doña Merilda typically saw between two and five patients a day, most of whom are neighborhood children brought by their mothers. She charged 5 Q (US$0.70) for adults and 3 Q (US$0.43) for children, which she sometimes accepted in the equivalent value of eggs, dried beans, or other staple goods. Her fees as a healer supplemented her income as a weaver. I have gotten know Doña Merilda well over years of afternoon conversations when she has described her treatments and occasionally allowed me to observe her with a patient.

Most of Doña Merilda treatments for childhood diarrhea involve a combination of herbs, packaged pharmaceuticals, and Catholic prayer. When a child was overheated, Doña Merilda used an egg passed over the body, along with recitation of an "Our Father" and an "Ave Maria" to draw the heat out. She said that red diarrhea is always "hot" and must be treated by cooling the stomach down with a cool drink like Seven-Up. For diarrhea caused by cold or excess air in the stomach, she massaged the stomach with oil to make the air come out. For "cold" diarrhea, she also made an herbal drink from rue (*Ruta graveolens*) leaves and Alka-Seltzer in water that removes excess air and warms the stomach.

The third critical category of diarrhea, according to Doña Merilda, consists of more serious cases caused by worms, which are more common in the rainy season from May to September. She told me, "There is always diarrhea when the rain comes; it doesn't matter how careful you are. For this I use a natural medicine called pericon [*Tagetes lucida*]. I give them pericon with two 'Santamicinas' [acetaminophen] boiled in water with mint. This usually cures the rainy-season diarrhea from worms." Dissecting these cases formed a major preoccupation for Doña Merilda in our discussions of childhood diarrhea—these were the cases that required tenacity and finesse as a healer.

In cases of diarrhea caused by worms, Doña Merilda focuses her attention on calming the worms and inducing them back into their sac. She told me that only in extremely rare cases do worms become so agitated that they leave the child's body either through the mouth or in the feces. In these cases, Doña Merilda feels that children should go to the health center because clearly something is "wrong on the inside" if the worms want to leave their home inside the body. On one occasion, I was able to observe one of Doña Merilda's more complex treatments for difficult cases of diarrhea caused by worms. A mother from the neighborhood brought her two-year-old son to see Doña Merilda because he had had diarrhea off and on for three weeks. She had taken her son to the health center the previous week but said that they had not given her anything "strong enough" to stop the diarrhea. Doña Merilda assured the mother that diarrhea is very common at her son's age and reminded her that it was the beginning of the rainy season, so diarrhea is bound to happen.

Doña Merilda made her assessment of the child's condition by laying him flat on a table in her living room, checking his eyes and skin, and examining the qualities of the diarrhea the diaper he had to start wearing again. She determined that his diarrhea was caused by a case of worms. Because the case had been persistent, she decided to apply a "stronger" treatment: she made a poultice of water boiled with a branch of an avocado tree, mint, and *epazote* (*Dysphania ambrosioides*) leaves. The resulting liquid was absorbed in a small rag that was then coated in cooking oil. The rag was placed on the center of the stomach over the navel and was secured in place by wrapping a length of cloth around the boy's midsection. Doña Merilda said an "Ave Maria" and sent the boy home, telling his mother to come back the next day so that she could check his progress. I was not present when the child was brought back to see Doña Merilda three days later, but she reported that his condition was much improved.

Doña Merilda told me that if a case became more serious or prolonged, she would add toasted white bread to the poultice placed over the patient's navel. She said, "Worms like bread, and they like oil. They can smell it down at the stomach, and it makes them want to go back down and get in their sac around the stomach." She also said that if she recognizes a difficult case of *empacho*, the best remedy is for the patient to drink a whole bottle of milk of magnesia. She felt that this "cleans every bad thing out of the stomach and calms the child down."[56] The final type of worm-induced diarrhea that Doña Merilda discussed with me was that resulting from *susto*, a fright or soul-loss. She said that when the soul became lost, it frightened the worms, which in turn made the patient have a stomachache. For this condition, which she said she treats only rarely and which I never witnessed, she must call the soul back through water placed in a bucket with a stick of incense and roses and say prayers. The soul reunites with the body, the worms return to their sac, and the condition is resolved.

The syncretism of healing systems both by healers like Doña Merilda and by patients using treatments from more than one source becomes clear in small villages like Panaj where options are more limited. There has been debate about the degree to which local or traditional healers continue to be used in Guatemala, with one study of childhood illness showing virtually no use of healers and another arguing that local healers continue to play a key role in treatment-seeking for Guatemalan Maya populations.[57] Local healers are syncretic practitioners within an increasingly pluralistic health care environment. They can be quietly consulted close to home and with lower financial barriers. In fact, their accessibility may obscure their continued presence and influence on health-seeking behaviors. Local healers may be invisible to researchers that only ask about them. It reminds me of the time I was helping facilitate a focus group on child nutrition in a rural Maya community. The participants kept listing foods but, even after several prompts, did not mention corn tortillas. I asked about this staple food so central to Maya identity, and everyone started laughing—of course they eat tortilla! But to mention it was like mentioning the air they breathe. I think that describes how many view local healers—of course they are present in rural communities as sources of advice and traditional remedies, it goes without saying. As mothers navigate treatment-seeking for children, local healers help not just with remedies but with advice on how to choose among other health care options that may be needed.

Paying for Care in Rural Communities

As Doña Merilda's example in Comalapa illustrates, community-based healers continue to be important sources of health-seeking. While her practice centered on natural remedies and spiritual healing, other local healers combine their role as healers and medicine sellers, offering an in-community option for the purchase of manufactured remedies. These healers and medicine sellers create more direct bridges to the fee-for-service private sector that the neoliberal economy has favored. In the rural village of Panaj, in addition to two inactive government community health workers and a midwife, there is a woman who is a local healer and a man who is known as an injectionist. The injectionist was trained in the late 1980s as a community health worker, but he now works independently and purchases his supplies from a pharmacy in Comalapa. He makes a profit by charging 10 Q (US$1.43) per injection, the selection of which primarily includes acetaminophen, ibuprofen, and vitamin B12. He reported having only three or four customers per month, with about an equal mix of children and adults (primarily men) as patients. Mothers in the village told me that they would consult the injectionist for a child with a high fever, cough, and cold, but no mother said they would use the injectionist for a child with diarrhea.

Apart from women relatives, Lety, the local healer, was the person most frequently consulted on the health conditions of children in Panaj. Lety's role in the community as a healer is interesting and indicative of the syncretism that has occurred across market-driven health sectors. Although she is most commonly referred to as a healer (*curandera*), people in the village also called Lety a pharmacist and a community health worker, despite the fact that she has no formal training as a CHW. These distinctions are not particularly useful to the residents of Panaj; rather, of primary importance is the fact that they see Lety as a local source of health care provision and advice.

Lety performs a few traditional healing practices, such as passing an egg over the body to remove excess heat, and she sells biomedical remedies from her shop window (figure 4.2). The small shop, attached to her house

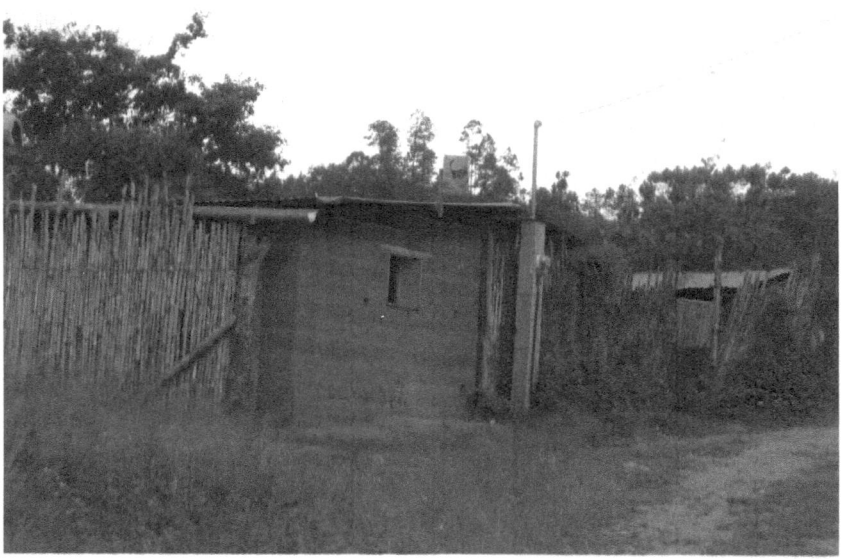

Figure 4.2
Local healer's shop window in Panaj.

and open most mornings and afternoons at her convenience, sells sodas, chips, and candy and provides Lety's main source of income. At any given time, Lety's stock of medicines is very small: a few blister packs of acetaminophen, liquid children's acetaminophen, and cough syrup. She buys these products when she buys other stock for her shop in Comalapa and sells them at a high profit, since she is the only medicine seller in the village. However, unlike formal pharmacies, Lety will sell her medicines by the dose, which makes them an attractive option for the cash-poor, which is essentially everyone in the village.

As a respected, middle-aged woman who has raised her own children, Lety is a trusted source of advice for childhood illnesses, including diarrhea. While it obviously behooves her to recommend the treatments she offers, Lety occasionally recommends that a mother take a child into town to the health center. She told me that she thinks ORT is good for children with diarrhea and that she sometimes sells it in her shop. However, over the months that I visited her shop regularly, including the beginning of the rainy season when diarrhea is more common, she never had any ORT in stock. She also asserted that Coca-Cola combined with acetaminophen syrup is a good treatment for many cases of childhood diarrhea, which, of course, she does sell in her shop. While Lety makes money as a healer in Panaj, she is not viewed as an opportunist by her neighbors, and she frequently gives out casual advice for free (though typically to customers of the shop). Lety is a polymath who, without the continuous presence of other health services in the village, provides treatments across the traditional and biomedical sectors. She personifies the transition to the global neoliberal economy, in which health can be bought and sold, and also local agency in how to engage with monetized health-seeking. Perhaps most importantly, Lety helps women make choices not just about the treatments she has in her shop but also the options available beyond the village that they may need to seek for their sick children.

Heggenhougen remarked on the health care situation in the Chimaltenango Department in the 1970s: "The [Kaqchikel] were faced with the classic double dilemma of having been influenced enough by the ladino world to doubt the powers of traditional curing practices and of finding western medicine inaccessible."[58] In the intervening years, the gap between traditional healing practices and formal biomedical services has been bridged with a complex array of products and services available in the marketplace—a bridge that buckles and gives way each time a person has no money. Perhaps the most remarkable feature of market-driven health care is that its elements—private clinics, pharmaceuticals, and local healers—are not used in isolation. Rather, treatment-seeking occurs across these options, according to affordability and accessibility. The affirmation of decision-making autonomy through the purchase of these products is encouraging in some ways: individual empowerment, social enterprise, and local profit-sharing, to name a few. However, with each purchase made, individuals assume a burden, perhaps construed as choice, for provisioning their own health care and absolve the government of its promise to enact health as a human right.

The Failures of "Free"

Returning to the exploration of diarrheal treatment-seeking and ORT use in Chimaltenango, we must consider its primary alternatives: waiting for an episode of diarrhea to pass and, if it does not, seeking strong treatments of antibiotics or IV fluids. Preference for antibiotics among poor Indigenous populations is closely tied to the issue of access to formal health care. These biomedical commodities create a cultural hegemony over less expensive treatments for diarrhea because of their associations with higher economic standards of living and quality of care. Knowledge of appropriate use of and access to these treatments is distributed unequally across Guatemalan society based on the elite structures and groups advantaged by the neoliberal economy. As we saw in chapter 3, access to the government health system is guaranteed to be free but ancillary costs, such as travel, lost work, and payments for tests and supplies, means that "free" care is never really free. Here I explore the implications of the cost spectrum on care and question the neoliberal notion that choice is necessarily advantageous.

We know that the distribution of goods and services across any society, particularly one with high socioeconomic disparities, as in Guatemala, is not equal. As one Kaqchikel Maya mother said in Acatenango, "We just give them [children with diarrhea] home remedies and nothing else because we have no money to take them to a specialist. It is just God and the home remedies." Ichiro Kawachi and Lisa Berkman observe that the settlement patterns of different socioeconomic groups and the placement of public goods and services are often a primary form of both overt and covert discrimination.[59] The distribution of health services in Chimaltenango discriminates against poor rural communities, which is to say the Kaqchikel Maya; this discrimination results in limited access to (appropriate use of) ORT. In examining ORT, Patrick Kenya and colleagues write, "The ultimate use of ORT is a function of its socio-cultural acceptability, the appropriateness of use, its availability and its accessibility."[60]

During a focus group discussion, a mother from a community of Acatenango summed up the issues of accessing effective health care in her community:

> Look, lady, here many things are needed. . . . Everybody here is poor, therefore we are needy. There's not ORS at the health center; we have to buy it at pharmacies. If we go to the health center, they only give us a little jar of acetaminophen and we are sent home. We can get ORS at the pharmacies, but they are very expensive, and we have no money to buy it. There are medicines, but we cannot afford them.

These frustrations were echoed time and time again by mothers trying to access health services for their children. I was repeatedly told of trips to health posts and government pharmacies that were out of ORT or simply closed without warning. When mothers did access health services, they were often dissatisfied with the level of attention they received from health staff. As described in chapter 3, when distances to health centers are far, mothers tend to wait longer to take their children for medical attention when the condition is perceived as a nonemergency, as in many cases of diarrhea. In the context of Chimaltenango, distances are difficult to traverse by foot because of the steep terrain. Mothers living in rural villages must often walk considerable distances to the nearest health post while carrying their sick child. Transportation to the nearest town from villages can be very limited. For example, in Panaj, on the twice-weekly market days, a handful of trucks bring paying passengers into town. Even in a car, the journey over rough, unpaved roads is difficult with a sick child.

Beyond the distances and difficulty in traversing rough terrain to reach a health care facility, the journeys to seek treatment for sick children take time away from mothers who have work they must accomplish within the household and in the fields to ensure the health and survival of their families. Particularly in instances where a husband or partner is away working in wage labor, women are responsible for maintaining and harvesting the crops that will help sustain them throughout the year. Women in this situation are particularly disinclined to make a tedious, sometimes expensive journey to a health care facility, only to receive unsatisfactory care. A mother with many young children must either manage the trip with all of them or find a relative or neighbor to look after the others while she is away.

The poor in Chimaltenango frequently cited not only distance but also money as a reason for delayed treatment-seeking for children with diarrhea. As one focus group participant from a village outside of Acatenango said, "If we had money, we would take the children to a doctor, because when we have money we take them sooner. [We] take them to a private hospital to a specialist, where they cure them faster and better." During conversations about diarrhea treatment-seeking, many informants indicated their perception that private health care is of a higher standard than the government health service. Yet few rural Indigenous caregivers have access to these health resources. Private doctors are primarily accessible for residents of urban areas, whose children, by virtue of their family's higher socioeconomic status and better living conditions, experience fewer bouts of diarrhea.

We have seen the preference for expensive ORS solutions rather than free or low-cost ORS packets because it is easier to get children to drink them and also because of the social status they convey. We have also learned that having a child with diarrhea outside of expected seasons and developmental milestones is a source of embarrassment for mothers. It follows, then, that poor mothers would be unable to afford "prestige" treatments like bottled ORS or a private doctor, but they are also likely to be reluctant to call public attention to their child's diarrhea by asking for a loan to seek treatment.

If families do pay and take the time to travel to a health care facility, they want to be compensated for their efforts with a treatment perceived as strong and effective. ORT is not perceived as such a treatment, and more interventionist treatments like antibiotics and IV fluids are highly valued. A doctor on the mobile health team in Comalapa remarked, "People here don't accept ORT very well. They want something more heroic [stronger], such as an injection or more expensive pills, like antibiotics. They don't like the little envelopes much. We are always talking with them to change their minds." It stands to reason that if there is but one limited opportunity to access the health care system for a case of diarrhea, a concerned parent would desire a treatment they feel sure will work the first time. In fact, mobile doctors who work with rural communities believe that mothers often exaggerate their reports of symptoms in their children to prompt a more powerful treatment. One mother, whose child was hooked up to IV fluids in the departmental hospital, told me, "This is the best cure you can get. This is the only thing that works." What may be classified as unnecessary or "irrational" use of more invasive interventions like IVs or pharmaceuticals like antibiotics in resource-constrained contexts such as Guatemala makes sense given limited accessibility of health care.[61]

Purchasing "Strong Medicine"

We have seen that many barriers delay care-seeking for childhood diarrhea, but there is a preference for strong treatment when care is sought. If waiting-and-seeing ultimately leads mothers to having to act, it stands to reason that they would choose the strongest treatment they can afford, as in the example of Josefina, a young mother of two small children in Panaj. Josefina's husband grows broccoli and blackberries as cash crops on his modest plots of land in addition to the family's subsistence foods of maize and beans. Her family does not live in the best or the worst house in the village, and they are broadly representative of an average family's economic condition in Panaj. Josefina's youngest son, nineteen-month-old Reynaldo, became sick with diarrhea at the start of the rainy season in May. As a doting mother who prides herself on being "modern" in the care of her children, Josefina started to keep a more watchful eye on him and swaddled him up in a sling on her back, even though he had grown too large to comfortably be carried all day. She also made him cups of the powdered *atol* corn porridge provided by the mobile health teams, and she became more concerned when Reynaldo, usually a voracious eater, was uninterested in it and other foods.

After a couple of days, Josefina carried Reynaldo the thirty to forty-five minutes to the nearest health post, but it was closed. She decided to return home and wait to see if the diarrhea would clear up on its own. When the next market day came around and Josefina needed to go into town in Comalapa to sell some of her weavings, she decided to leave Reynaldo, who by this point had had diarrhea for five days, at home with her mother-in-law to spare him the exhaustion of the trip to town. All day, she fretted over how Reynaldo might be doing, and using a significant portion of her earnings, Josefina bought a packet of antibiotics before returning home. The purchase involved intense negotiation with the man vending pharmaceuticals at an open-air table in the market. She described her son's condition, and he suggested two packets of an antiparasitic. Josefina could not afford those, so eventually she and the vendor settled on the antibiotics, which he assured her would take care of Reynaldo's diarrhea. In the face of a shortage of medicines or the funds to buy them, a customer can either look elsewhere for the desired product or reformulate their ideas of what constitutes an effective treatment to coincide with what is readily available.[62] Belief in which treatment will create the desired health outcome is shaped by supply and purchasing power.

Over the next three days, Josefina gave Reynaldo all of the antibiotics (amoxicillin), but to no avail. Reynaldo was still sick, and she had spent all she could afford. Fortunately, the mobile health team made a visit to the village on the third day of Reynaldo's antibiotics, and Josefina took him out to see the doctor. The doctor examined him, finding him feverish and with slight dehydration, and asked Josefina what she had been giving him. When she told him about the antibiotics, he became irate, poking her in the shoulder and loudly chiding her that she had probably made Reynaldo sicker. He told her that antibiotics are not good for very small children and can make the stomach hurt more in the case of diarrhea. He gave her one packet of ORS and told her to continue to keep Reynaldo hydrated, and he assured her that this would make Reynaldo better.

Reynaldo did get better a few days after the doctor's visit. Josefina mixed up the one ORS packet with boiled water in a pot on her cooking fire and tried to give him sips of it from a cup. He did not like it, and she stored the remainder of the solution in the pot, covered with a plate, for several days. Josefina was left feeling relieved that Reynaldo got better but frustrated and angered by how the doctor spoke to her. She told me that she tries to do everything right for her children, and she wishes she could give them good medicine like rich people do. That is what she felt she was doing by purchasing the expensive antibiotics, and she still felt that they had helped Reynaldo get better. "These doctors, they don't know everything. Us mothers learn what works with our kids," she said. She said that she had done everything possible for Reynaldo's sickness, and she would do the same things again in the future.

The phenomenon of self-prescribed medicines, primarily antibiotics, is common across Guatemala. As the mobile doctor warned Josefina, antibiotics are very dangerous for small children, particularly in large doses. This can be especially hazardous for young children in Chimaltenango, who experience frequent bouts of diarrhea during weaning and while learning to walk. Their parents often perceive "strong" packaged medicines to be the best treatment available for a persistent case of diarrhea, and they can receive many unprescribed rounds of antibiotics. Strong medicine comes with more than economic costs. Overuse of antibiotics in children can lead to organ damage and, if not correctly prescribed, a worsening of the bout of diarrhea by upsetting the natural balance of bacteria in the gut.[63]

Misuse and overuse of antibiotics are concerns for the health sector in Guatemala, and the Ministry of Public Health and Social Assistance created new regulations in 2019 for the storage, prescription control, and dispensation of antibiotics.[64] However, in practice, implementation of these new regulations has been slow, and pharmaceuticals continue to be widely available for purchase in pharmacies and markets. A conversation that I had with a UNICEF Guatemala official gave me insight to this ambivalent government approach, recognizing the need for greater regulation yet not taking steps toward meaningful implementation. He commented, "People expect to be able to buy antibiotics for themselves and their children, and they believe in them. The government cannot provide health consultations for everyone, so it is best that people are able to choose what they want to use." His point was that national dissatisfaction with public goods and services would prevent the government from implementing new regulatory measures, as this would be seen as impinging on the population's already limited access to health care. If the government cannot make good on the promise of free, accessible care, as guaranteed as a human right by Guatemalan law, it will do little to regulate the freedom of choice of individuals within the health care marketplace.

Aspirational Care and the Role of Short-Term Medical Missions

As we have seen, more costly care brings prestige, as in the examples of Omnilife and other private sector offerings. Health care associated with foreigners also brings prestige and, for some, a vital source of care that would otherwise be out of reach. Here I describe short-term medical missions

(STMMs) as part of the constellation of on-the-ground treatment-seeking options. STMMs are a health care model in which health providers, students, and other volunteers travel internationally to deliver free or very low-cost medical care, dentistry, or surgery for a period ranging from a few days up to two years.[65] Many STMMs also undertake water, sanitation, and hygiene education. Over the years, I have seen STMM groups conduct education sessions ranging from a thoughtful information session on use of ORT with clear visual aids to a bizarre toothbrushing demonstration on a big set of fake teeth.

Most STMMs in Guatemala, of which there are hundreds per year, are one to two weeks in length and range in organizational sophistication from transnational NGOs with permanent in-country staff to small groups of independent foreigners. You practically cannot fly from the United States to Guatemala without sharing a plane with an STMM team—they are easy to spot with their huge luggage and matching T-shirts. Although STMMs bring an endlessly shifting stream of providers, they have come to form a durable part of the Guatemalan health care landscape, contributing to a philanthropic sector that bridges gaps in the public and private health care sectors. While childhood diarrhea is often too episodic to appear exactly when an STMM is in town, STMMs frequently provide primary care and basic health and hygiene education. STMMs are a key element of the Guatemalan health care system and feature prominently on the rural poor's mental map of possible resources.

In Guatemala, STMMs desire to reach populations that cannot afford private care for conditions for which public sector care is unavailable or has a long waitlist. In doing so, STMMS try to provide care that would otherwise be inaccessible; however, they introduce some critical challenges to quality of care and health equity.[66] Because foreign volunteers often have little cultural or linguistic concordance with their local patients, clear and accurate communication can be difficult.[67] STMMs generate ancillary costs for patients (such as for food, housing, travel, lab tests), which again excludes or unfairly burdens the poorest care-seekers, although some of the larger NGO-coordinated STMMs provide transportation and housing.[68] Scholarship on STMMs has tended to focus on the experiences of volunteer providers rather than the patients and recipient communities.[69] Among volunteer providers and organizers of STMMs, global research has found the pervasive idea that some care is better than no care, leading to issues with quality and safety of care. Perhaps the most enduring challenge of STMMs is the difficulty in providing adequate post-operative follow-up care or care for chronic conditions, since the visiting foreign providers are gone by the time complications may arise.[70]

Ultimately, STMMs generate parallel health delivery systems that serve crucial immediate needs but do not meaningfully contribute to durable health system strengthening. STMMs creates additional regulatory burdens for the recipient country to assess qualifications of foreign providers and provide oversight of their work—a burden that often goes unfulfilled. Guatemala has legal regulations for STMMs, requiring that groups be registered, that all foreign providers file their professional licenses with the College of Doctors and Surgeons of Guatemala, and that they be supervised by a licensed Guatemalan provider during their mission.[71] While registration requirements have been updated and better implemented in recent years, significant gaps in oversight on the scope and quality of care given by foreign providers persist.

I had a conversation on a flight from Guatemala with a veterinarian returning to the United States following a weeklong service trip. He proudly told me of the surgeries he had performed within Indigenous communities in the highlands—on people! When I questioned his confidence in being able ability to safely provide surgeries, he shrugged and said with a smile, "I guess I'm better than nothing for those people." Something is often far more dangerous than nothing, and the idea that a different standard of safety and quality could be permissible in poor Guatemalan communities than in US or other high-income contexts is deeply disturbing. While many foreign providers visit Guatemala each year and provide safe, high-quality care in appropriate health care settings, the variability among STMMs as a mechanism for delivering care feels like a high-stakes lottery.

Individuals within communities who seek care from STMMs are typically not able to adjudicate the quality of care of foreign medical teams—how could they possibly? So, individuals rely on their social networks and the received wisdom of word-of-mouth advice to find out about available STMM care and experiences of the quality of that care. STMMs use a variety of recruitment methods to find patients for visiting medical teams, ranging from having staff enroll patients in advance to placing radio advertisements to just showing up and putting out a sign. Word spreads among community networks, and care-seekers serendipitously connect with an STMM that can care for their particular health issue. The problem, of course, is that the human right to health should not rely on serendipity.

The free or low-cost care of STMMs does come with a price. Recipients of STMM care by foreign providers are expected to be grateful.[72] In a study of patient and caregiver experiences of surgical care from STMMs, my colleagues and I found that even when serious complications arose following surgery, recipients were reluctant to express critiques or describe negative experiences. One mother whose child had received surgical care and then faced life-threatening complications after the foreign providers had left the community asked us to stop recording the interview when she described this harrowing experience. The moment she signaled for the voice-recorder to be turned back on, she expressed her thanks to the foreign providers for their free surgical care.[73] The STMM model of care generates problematic gratitude. Recipients of care are expected to express gratitude, and the coordinating local and transnational NGOs must demonstrate both gratitude and "impact" to keep foreign providers motivated to continue volunteering.[74] Just as low- and middle-income countries are beholden to high-income countries for foreign aid and must accede to their terms, recipients of STMM care are supposed to be grateful no matter what happens.

While STMMs offer an option where the health services themselves are either free or very low cost, they contribute to the notion that private health care is more valuable than public sector care—and that care provided by foreigners must somehow be even more valuable still. Just like the Behrhorst Clinic trades on being the "hospital del gringo," care from foreign visiting medical teams is highly prized and reinforces neocolonial relationships. Within rural Maya communities, word of their availability spreads fast and adds to the confusing array of imperfect options among which care-seekers must choose. The neoliberal values of individual responsibility and self-reliance are entrenched even within "free" care in the philanthropic sector, with some STMMs even requesting "symbolic payments" so that recipients "value" the care they receive. Health becomes a commodity you can purchase rather than a human right meant for all.

Conclusion

"When you have money, you can buy anything, and when you don't, you can't," observed a mother in Panaj speaking about health care for her children. Within the vacuum created by a dearth of government health services, private health services and supplies have flourished. Health becomes something that you can choose to buy in the marketplace of care, and continuing centuries of default exclusion, it is unattainable by the Indigenous poor. While market-driven health services—from private clinics to marketplace (quasi)pharmaceuticals to the philanthropic sector—provide options from which to choose, they also serve to absolve the government of its duty of care and underpin an abdication of the right to health. Regulation of providers, pharmaceuticals, supplements, marketplace vendors, and foreign medical teams creates further burdens on an already overstretched, under-resourced government health system and is inconsistently implemented.

The trend toward the commodification of health and market-based models of health care system grew in low- and middle-income countries alongside the economic and political forces of globalization.[75] Globalization has created new participants in cash economies, and consequently, it has created new consumers and shaped the desires that pattern consumption. In Guatemala, as in much of the majority world, packaged pharmaceutical products, ORS solutions among them, are the aspirational vanguard of biomedicine and highly valued as symbols of progress. This, in turn, leads to a perception of health and health services as limited goods, available only to those with purchasing power. In terms of neoliberal economic rationality, the preference for costly and prestigious health treatments can seem irrational. Yet, as Salmaan Keshavjee observes, "In neoliberal terms, individual choices about purchasing goods and services in the private market without so-called government interference constitute 'freedom.'"[76] Poor, Maya communities in Guatemala have faced decades of brutal exclusion from social, economic, and political participation and centuries of marginalization. In this light, the small doses of freedom bought through health-seeking seem like a way to escape the impositions of the government and its health system. But within the neoliberal health care landscape, choice is an illusory proxy for accessible care, and price is a deceptive proxy for quality.

High-cost goods and services, like packaged pharmaceuticals, create a cultural hegemony because of their associations with high-income lifestyles and perceptions of quality of care.[77] The movement of goods sparked by globalization and codified through our neoliberal capitalist system has led to privatization and the reliance on public-private partnerships for the distribution of social goods.[78] Supply chains mean security in our contemporary global economy, and these supply chains are controlled by high-income countries globally and the wealthy elite within countries. The flow of social goods—including health resources and services—through supply chains to the poor of the majority world is intermittent and inadequate. As the poor residents of Chimaltenango are acutely aware, the commodities of biomedicine and knowledge of how to access biomedical care are not equally distributed around the globe or within societies. Ulf Hannerz has observed of other high-prestige cultural phenomena that while the elite are exposed to new resources, including knowledge, and are able to take advantage of the resultant economic and political opportunities, the poor receive only filtered, partial knowledge and limited access to resources.[79] The same unequal patterns of access to knowledge and resources occur for health-seeking. The neoliberal health care landscape is constantly in flux, so knowledge of how to navigate it successfully has a short half-life favoring the wealthy and well-connected and leaving the poor lost as it decays.

Members of Maya communities use the health system on their own terms, with some rejecting it as a representation of state interference while others argue for the expansion of services in their communities. The unequal distribution of the knowledge and commodities generates and perpetuates systemic inequalities and structural violence. A false freedom is generated by the pluralistic care landscape in Guatemala, which implies that hard work and serendipity are prerequisites for individuals to attain the human right to health supposedly guaranteed by one's humanity and affirmed by the Guatemalan constitution. The freedom to choose among available options is foreclosed for many by racism, social isolation, and economic disadvantage. Exerting the agency of choice in the Guatemalan health landscape can be exhausting, as products, goods, and services quickly come and go. Within a community of limited economic capital, individuals must draw on the social capital of their networks to mobilize the knowledge and resources required for treatment-seeking.[80] The confusion and burdens that choices create for care-seekers in neoliberal health systems are part of the hidden underbelly of global health—in which the neoliberal marketplace is unquestioned on its compatibility with the right to health. The structures of global health and development aid that channel the flow of biomedical knowledge and products and their inherent power imbalances are further explored next in chapter 5.

5 Global Guidelines, Local Realities: Complexities of Global Health

> Programs come and go. They lose excitement. But the people, we are always here, always the same. The next thing comes along, and we don't pay it too much attention. We know it will go the way of others, so people sometimes take what they can and forget about it.
>
> —community leader, village community of Acatenango

Ceci and I were chatting in the street when the truck came around the corner, scattering the waiting clusters of women and kids and easing to a stop in front of the nongovernmental organization (NGO) office (figure 5.1). The dry season dust it kicked up smarted in our eyes and dried up conversation. We had been talking about the NGO, formed as a transnational organization to eradicate poverty through education, funded through US donors, and implemented by program staff in Guatemala. Ceci felt that the program was "one of the good ones" because they gave good incentives for attending programs. It was with anticipation of these incentives that women followed the program staff into the local office in the front room of a house in Acatenango, filing into child-sized chairs to listen to how to keep their kids healthy and able to attend school. Heat and lassitude stifled the room, and heads drooped as staff droned on about handwashing, illustrated by cartoon drawings on posters. Finally, the session came to an end, and everyone went outside to the tailgate of the NGO truck to receive a box containing a bag of rice, a bag of dried black beans, a bottle of oil, and a sack of sugar. The normalcy of smiles and conversation returned to the street as the group spilled out of the room to claim their rewards. For Ceci, it was worth it.

Ceci had told me, "You can't count on programs like this, but it's good to get whatever things they give out when you can." As a stay-at-home mother

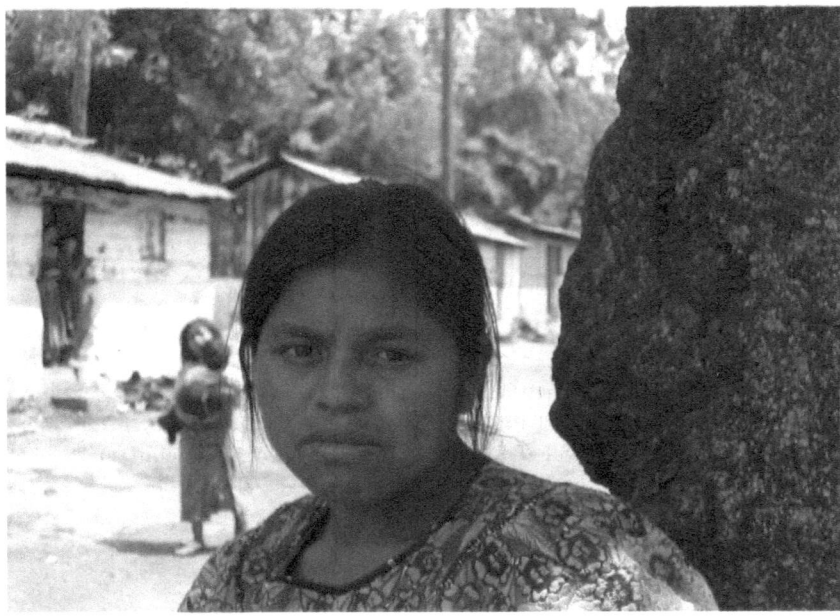

Figure 5.1
Mother on an Acatenango coffee plantation.

with four kids, Ceci was always looking for opportunities to supplement
the income of her husband from the coffee cooperative and to improve the
options for her school-age children. She told me that she would sign up for
any programs that came along. She remembered how another NGO used to
operate a child sponsorship program in the community to pay for school
supplies and provide tutoring; she began giggling as she recalled how much
her oldest son had hated having to write letters to his sponsor in the United
States. Ceci told me that her son had disliked sitting still and having to carefully copy out the scripted letter in English, but she said it was good for him
to "practice gratitude." I, on the other hand, remembered seeing the ads
for child sponsorship programs on television when I was growing up, their
stark and culpably evocative images of child poverty making me feel guilty
about my after-school snack and cartoons.

Ceci has practiced gratitude throughout her life as she has navigated the
opportunities for health-seeking and improved education for her family.
Yet Ceci's gratitude feels compulsory—an expectation of the NGOs who
dole out bits of the wealth of others. She chooses to participate, but the

limited options for health-seeking in her community entangle her in the well-worn tropes of how a recipient of the largess of others should act—that you should take what you can get and be grateful for it. The problematic gratitude expected of Ceci—giving up her time, sitting in tiny chairs, nodding along to instructions she cannot follow because they are so at odds with her material reality—pervades global health and development. This problematic gratitude exemplifies the asymmetries in global health and the unequal position the poor and marginalized hold in a neoliberal health care landscape.

This chapter moves from a focus on individual choices and actions within the fragmented, pluralistic Guatemalan health care system to consider the global health and development structures that have helped create this system. In Guatemala, as elsewhere in the majority world, the global health and development workforce, local and foreign, NGO and government alike, confront burnout and a sense of futility. I assert that the multiplicity and lack of coordination of health and development programming leads to an active inertia for health system strengthening, where despite a great deal of activity, little substantial, sustainable change is achieved. Expenditures of material and human resources that fail to create change are not just programmatic failures, but they cause harm by abetting entrenched inequalities. Guatemalans like Ceci, targeted by various global health and development efforts, have become jaded—they take what they can from new programs with the knowledge those programs will soon be gone and replaced by others. These systemic failures are not unique to Guatemala, and global health must reckon with unequal global (neo)colonial socioeconomic and political power dynamics to build systems of equity in their stead. In an era when global health and development funding is driven by the disease-specific goals and benchmarks set by powerful private donors and the governments of wealthy nations, we must also broaden our scope to address the underlying determinants of health, both physical and social. Despite these challenges, I believe we can identify pressure points within global health and development structures to move toward lasting change and effective collaboration with local communities.

Power and Positionality in Global Health, Development, and Humanitarian Enterprises

Global health and development structures are pluralistic and complex. Different actors promote their own varied agendas, and trends in key issues and strategies are ever-changing. At an anthropology conference, I once received a "more of a comment than a question" pointing out that global health, development, and humanitarianism are "entirely different fields because they have different literatures." Yes, they do! But with all due respect to my academic colleagues, it does not matter to Ceci which literature *we* use to frame *her* experiences of health and development programs in rural Guatemala. A wise colleague on a project in Rwanda once asked me, "When does the humanitarian emergency end and development begin? We are always living in a slow emergency."[1] As we will explore, global health builds on a long, problematic history of colonial health enterprises. Global health intersects with development sector efforts, and the umbrella of development institutions casts a wide shadow across economic and so-called human development to support durable change. For its part, the humanitarian aid sector is shaped to respond to crisis and emergency situations, but as my Rwandan colleague pointed out, the time frames and remits of the humanitarian response can grow blurry. Global health, development, and humanitarian aid sectors are deeply commingled on the ground, though the international financial structures and organizational missions that support them may diverge. In practice, it is often a shared, highly skilled set of local experts, providers, and implementation teams that do the operational work of global health, development, and humanitarian aid.

All global health, development, and humanitarian aid interventions have an underlying ideological justification for outsiders to intervene in specific ways. Interventions are never neutral.[2] Development programs, controlled by high-income countries, get to define what "development" is. Though contemporary global health is centered on the ideological justification of social justice, global health interventions are shaped by the moral values of our dominant global neoliberal geopolitical system.[3] The challenges taken up by humanitarianism are a foreign imaginary. Foreign-led groups decide to focus on some problems and ignore others, setting the agendas of humanitarian enterprises including global health.[4] Within countries, this means that governments do not always get to choose priority sectors for intervention and that people like Ceci do not get to choose who or what shows up in a truck in their community.

As we saw with the foreign teams on short-term medical missions in chapter 4, the good intentions of the humanitarian impulse can lead to bad outcomes. The entanglements of compassion and politics in humanitarianism is centered on relationships of giving and their potential for imbalances.[5] As Ilana Feldman and Miriam Ticktin state, "Humanitarianism is produced at the intersection between sentiment and material inequality," setting forth inherently asymmetrical relationships of solidarity and compassion embedded in our contemporary reckonings of humanitarianism.[6] Global health has drawn on an increasingly globalized value system—economic, political, and social—that has come to rely on contradictory ideals of humanitarianism for enacting human rights.[7] Yet humanitarianism is rooted in our human capacity for care and caregiving.[8] It is how we channel and shape that capacity—individually and collectively—in global health that matters.

Despite good intentions and the human capacity for care, an aura of frustration and futility looms over many development workers, local and foreign, NGO and government alike in Guatemala, as elsewhere in the majority world. Development efforts in Guatemala face two key challenges: first, the corrupt and weak government does not prioritize necessary infrastructure and resources, and second, a lack of coordination among NGOs and the philanthropic sector leads to a chaos of overlapping projects. The big picture of global health and development work is critical to understanding how care-seeking pathways available within communities are shaped and how global health interventions like oral rehydration therapy (ORT) are set in motion. Changes in global health paradigms since the early 2000s, set in large part by major funders, have led to preferences for projects with finite, measurable outcomes. ORT does not easily fit this mold; as we have seen, cases of childhood diarrheal disease and use of ORT in the home are difficult to count. While ORT programs in Chimaltenango and elsewhere are eroding, diarrhea remains a critical child health issue. Global health and the challenges it chooses to address are shaped by donor-driven trends, colonial legacies, and the contemporary neoliberal political economy.

Paradigm Shifts in Global Health and Development: Neoliberalism Is the New Colonial Medicine

During the colonial land grabs of the eighteenth century, wealthy European nations further capitalized on the extractive wealth of the age of conquest amassed over the previous centuries. The system of global peonage set up during this period persists today, with wealthy countries extracting natural resources and human labor from the majority world. The bonds of conquest and colonialism have a stranglehold on our contemporary neo-liberal economy; as Emmanuel Wallerstein articulated in world systems theory, the "core" countries continue to dominate and dictate the terms of global economic and political relationships to "peripheral" countries.[9] The extraction of resources creates profit for the high-income countries, and the resultant need in majority world countries leads to indebtedness and weak positioning in the global political economy (figure 5.2). The unjustly enriched countries are then positioned to "save" the countries they have impoverished on their own terms and when they choose to do so.

During the nineteenth century, rife with racialized pseudoscience and eugenics, the colonial notion of the "white man's burden" took hold.[10] This was a paternalistic and racist doctrine asserting that colonized peoples were incapable of governing themselves, so guidance was needed to civilize and Christianize them. Global health has its roots in the colonial medicine of this era. Colonial tropical medicine was first and foremost concerned with the health of colonizers carrying out the work of extraction; a begrudging secondary concern was to maintain a healthy workforce among the local population.[11] Following World War II, the victors of the war, dominated by the

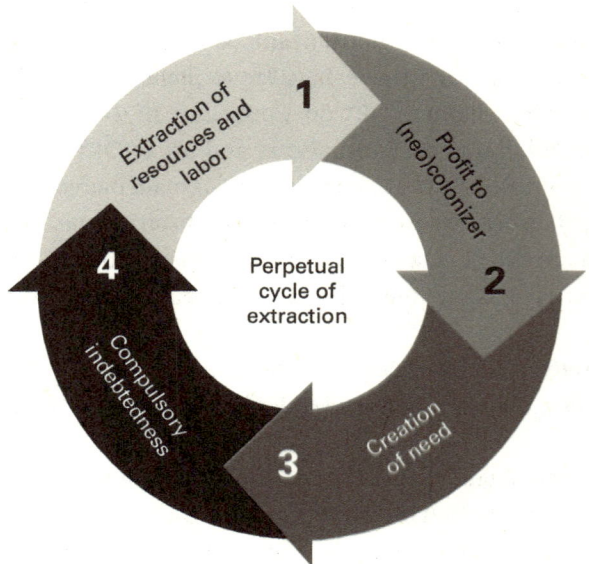

Figure 5.2
Cycle of extraction from the majority world to high-income countries.

United States, led a flurry of global institution-building and the codification of human rights. Global health efforts were known as international health during this period and emphasized technocratic, vertical programs. Newly minted international organizations and multilateral government agencies, including the World Health Organization (WHO), directed interventions down through national and local levels of government.[12] The international health approach was effective in targeting specific diseases, such as the success of the smallpox eradication campaign, but it became muddled as an approach to global health intervention since multiple uncoordinated projects were often operating and competing for resources within the same geographic areas.

As a result, the global health paradigm swung from disease-specific approaches toward an emphasis on community-based primary health care in the 1970s, with the goal of creating more horizontal, integrated approaches to global health.[13] During the 1970s, the WHO became increasingly active as a monitoring and interventionist agency worldwide. The 1978 Alma-Ata Declaration of WHO member states declared "Health for All by the Year 2000" as the unachievable but lofty goal of their collective efforts. It aimed for all people in all countries to have access to health care, including mental health and social services. The 1978 declaration provided the impetus for primary health care programs around the globe, and Guatemala was proudly represented at the Alma-Ata conference by the Behrhorst Clinic, showcasing its early model of training community health workers to deliver primary health care.[14]

Parallel to governmental global health institutions and structures, nongovernmental organizations emerged as key actors in the application of post–World War II human rights and increasingly engagement in global health. During the 1970s and 1980s, interest groups focused on humanitarian values began to wield real influence on policymakers. Within the US context, NGOs began to take a more concrete role in creating US foreign policy, which shaped the focus of foreign aid and global health packages around the world and, in particular, in Latin America.[15] Human rights and development actors coalesced in transnational advocacy networks that include "international and domestic NGOs, foundations, and some governmental and intergovernmental officials who share collective understandings and a collective identity with regard to human rights norms."[16]

Between 1973 and 1985, these human rights advocacy networks expanded and, in conjunction with states, built the international structure of human rights norms and their attendant development institutions. Health via access to health care came to be considered as a basic human right. Between 1973 and 1990, the majority of high-income countries adopted explicit bilateral and multilateral human rights policies.[17] These transnational advocacy networks created a global civil society in which nonstate actors gain influence by serving as alternate sources of information and services.[18] This is consistent with the shift to neoliberal economic policies through which private, nonstate actors come to replace an increasingly weak state. Paradoxically, NGO-provided information is often used to promote government accountability while NGO-provided services can enable government shirking of service responsibilities to citizens. Both are true in Guatemala.

The 1970s and 1980s push for primary health care as the strategy to achieve "Health for All" faltered. The Alma-Ata emphasis on primary health care struggled from the outset to achieve its goals, including in Guatemala, and the primary health care movement ultimately came under critique for serving as a justification for low-quality health care.[19] Particularly before the advent of high-quality mobile health technologies, "appropriate technology" was used as shorthand for inferior products and technologies created for use in low-resourced contexts. It was a widely used global health term rationalizing poor quality for poor populations.[20] Quick and dirty fixes for the provision of primary care were rife and, unsurprisingly, did not yield the hoped-for durable health system strengthening so desperately needed to achieve health for all. The primary care focus made it more difficult to show measurable results than the disease-focused approaches, and ultimately, metrics are what came to matter in global health.

The shift away from primary care and integrative approaches to global health back toward disease-specific, technocratic approaches began in earnest in the 1990s. At this point, contemporary global health structures were well-established, with multilateral government organizations, such as the WHO, and bilateral government organizations, like the US Agency for International Development, taking leadership of defining and channeling funding for priority areas. Transnational NGOs form a broad category that includes heavy hitters such as the Gates Foundation as well as smaller NGOs with a direct relationship between donor and recipient countries. While several large global NGOs have a presence in Guatemala, much of the NGO landscape is populated by smaller transnational NGOs that fundraise in the United States and deliver programs in Guatemala. Finally, at the base of the global health pyramid are local organizations—including government health systems and local NGOs. As we have seen in the pluralistic care landscape in Guatemala, these are the organizations that actually implement global health programming. They do not typically, however, decide what issues will be prioritized or how implementations are designed. Public-private partnerships are built across all tiers of the contemporary global health structure. For example, we have seen this in the delivery of health care in Guatemala, where the government has relied on both local NGOs to deliver health care and foreign providers and transnational NGOs to bridge gaps in the coverage they offer.

Primary care-focused efforts were diffuse and difficult to measure, and as a result, global health priorities shifted back toward disease-focused and condition-specific programs that better aligned with a metric-driven political economy of global health. The Millennium Development Goals created umbrella global goals and a reporting structure across the United Nations (UN) system for the eradication of poverty and health promotion, with each member country setting specific targets for the 2000–2015 period.[21] The growing political and economic influence of bilateral government organizations and transnational NGOs also became apparent by the early 2000s. Efforts like the US President's Emergency Plan for AIDS Relief (PEPFAR), which provided unprecedented levels of funding for HIV/AIDS starting in 2003, concretized the shift toward disease-specific programming. The rise of the Gates Foundation in the 2000s furthered the philanthropic sector's influence in setting the global health agenda.[22]

With the renewed focus on disease-specific programs, global health evaluation became (even) more tightly focused on quantitative metrics—big funding programs need to yield impressive, quantifiable results to justify more funding.[23] And they have delivered! Even if imperfect, great strides were made during the period of the Millennium Development Goals in improving the health of global populations. The Sustainable Development Goals that followed have included the agreement of UN member states to try to achieve universal health coverage by 2030.[24] The Sustainable Development Goals, particularly the target for achieving universal health coverage, point toward more meaningful efforts at health systems strengthening and the integration of primary care–focused and disease-specific approaches. The ongoing Sustainable Development Goals have built on the progress and metric evaluation structures of the Millennium Development Goals, but aligning the metrics collected to clear indicators of (lasting) change is difficult.[25] Metrics and the accountability they can facilitate are vital tools in the contemporary global health ecosystem. However, they can lead to tunnel vision on what is important, encourage fudging of numbers to meet expectations (across all tiers of hierarchical reporting structures), and fall into the vertical program trap of working to achieve predetermined goals that do not map to improvements on the ground in communities.[26]

Over the past seventy years, global health has inarguably achieved great successes, from the elimination and eradication of some infectious diseases to the reduction of child mortality, in part thanks to ORT, and extended life expectancies globally. However, these gains have not been distributed equally. Of course not. Our contemporary system of global health structures and actors struggles to break free of the power dynamics of colonial relationships (as in figure 5.2). While the post–World War II era moved us from tropical medicine to the international health paradigm that has now become global health, we can also see the concomitant emergence of a bureaucratic global health elite of experts who have largely been from and represented the interests of high-income countries.[27] William Easterly's term "the tyranny of experts" is apt—the professionalization of the global health workforce across public, private, and philanthropic sectors has further perpetuated power inequalities in global health and enabled high-income countries to continue to set agendas and dominate leadership of the field.[28] Contemporary global health interventions are centered on social justice, but we have failed to apply this moral position to our own field. Asymmetrical power dynamics continue to shape global health structures and delivery, which only serves to maintain the status quo it purportedly fights against.

The spheres of influence of high-income countries within global health replicate (neo)colonial patterns, with European programmatic dominance in Africa and Asia and US dominance in Latin America. I will never forget attending a meeting in the UK Parliament on "neglected tropical diseases" to share interim data on a malaria project. After listening to all the progress and data, an older Member of Parliament sighed and remarked, "Oh, it was so much easier when we could just tell them what to do over there and make it happen." My jaw dropped—he said the quiet colonialism out loud! My shock was a sign of my own privilege, and I know my colleagues from the majority world have heard and lived this paternalistic attitude daily. Despite this vocal supporter of the colonial enterprise, I think global health has a workforce, thankfully increasingly inclusive of experts from majority world contexts, who want to make social justice and global health equity real. Our global health systems and neoliberal funding structures get in the way.

Buying Health: Who Pays in the Neoliberal Marketplace?

Critical global need for access to health care remains. At least half of the world's population still does not have full coverage of essential health services. About 100 million people are pushed into extreme poverty annually because of health care costs.[29] Growth in spending on health care is outpacing growth of gross domestic product (GDP) across countries globally, regardless of income level. However, high-income countries have the largest percentage of health care costs covered by government expenditures, and low-income countries have the largest percentage covered by out-of-pocket expenditures.[30]

Current global health spending is dominated by governments of high-income countries and a few key NGOs backed by philanthropic donors, among which the Gates Foundation commands unparalleled resources. Although donor funding in global health has been falling since 2014, donor spending still accounts for nearly 30 percent of health expenditures in low-income countries.[31] While the contributions of high-income countries are the primary source of funding in global health, contributions remain a very low proportion of high-income country budgets. For example, US foreign aid accounts for just above one percent of the annual government budget, inclusive of military assistance and national security work.[32] Financial contributions are tailored to further the donor's goals and the motivations that underpin them. Global health funders, government and NGO alike, need to see the impact of their investments and show the efficacy of their interventions. While data may not always drive their priority areas, they drive the assessment of "success." In order to understand how Ceci and others across Guatemala encounter global health programs, we must consider the drivers of foreign aid and development funding in Latin America.

Global Health and Development Funding in Latin America

During the 1990s, the Latin American region experienced a trend toward liberal democracy, which had the goal of promoting health care reform and breaking governments' habits of using access to health care as a means by which to extract political patronage. This trend focused new attention on the ability, capacity, and willingness of state agencies to implement changes in health policy. Few countries in the region have the resources to implement comprehensive health care reform, leading to patterns of distribution of (limited) resources that reflect social inequalities.[33] By the end of the 1990s, Latin America had become a major market for United States private health sector engagement, including insurance companies and health care maintenance organizations, emphasizing the regional turn to neoliberal health care in the past thirty years.[34] Privatization—both through for-profit health sector offerings and through philanthropic partnerships—became the default for government health systems with limited finances.

In Guatemala and throughout the region, health and development transnational advocacy networks form an important conduit for global health financing and government accountability. As described in chapter 3, global neoliberal development institutions like the International Monetary Fund and the World Bank set the terms for development loans and strategic areas for foreign investment. The Pan American Health Organization (PAHO), the regional branch of the WHO, is headquartered in Guatemala City, and a vast array of other bilateral government agencies and NGOs provide programming throughout the region. PAHO is the principal global health actor in Latin America, with country offices in twenty-seven of the thirty-five member nations in the Americas. The total estimated budget for the 2020–2021 fiscal year is $650 million, over half of which is raised through donor partners and the WHO.[35] Many bilateral government health and development organizations are active in the region. The US Agency for International Development (USAID) has a significant presence regionally and in Guatemala in particular. USAID often contracts implementation of programs to local organizations and builds partnerships with NGOs. However, acting on US interests and priorities, a vast proportion of USAID spending in Latin America goes toward countering narcotrafficking to US territory.

For my own part in these structures, I have read the reports, seen program statistics, and attended presentations from many of the global health and development institutions in Guatemala. I have primarily been funded by

US government research funds, institutional grants from my own university, and foundations, and I have mostly partnered with small local organizations on research and implementation work over the past fifteen years. So I was surprised when my office phone rang in Atlanta a few years ago, and it was a US government-led initiative, backed by the Interamerican Development Bank, to help address root causes of child migration. They wanted me to propose a project to help solve "push factors" for migration, such as poor access to health care. Now, I am very grateful and proud of the work I have been able to do in Guatemala, but I am scarcely the lynchpin that can magically fix the health system. I can only assume that they did a lot of googling in English to come across me. My efforts to connect and suggest Guatemalan health and civil society leaders as better points of contact went nowhere, and I declined to pursue the opportunity. It felt like I was living out neocolonial patterns and assumptions; it would be "easier" and yield "more measurable" results if a US academic could be the recipient of funding rather than a community organization that could actually do the work. Fundamentally, our systems must work better for the people they are meant to serve.

Neoliberal Health in Guatemala

NGOs, as we saw in chapters 3 and 4, have become vital actors within the Guatemalan health system, both participating in public-private partnerships and serving as safety nets for lapses of the public system. In the years since the internal armed conflict and the boom of foreign aid began in the mid-1990s, NGOs have proliferated—more than 10,000 NGOs are registered to operate in Guatemala, many with a mission related to poverty reduction or health.[36] At the same time, the Guatemalan government affirmed health as a human right and promised free health care for all. But, as we have seen from the experiences of Maya people and communities throughout this book, the government cannot fully deliver on this promise. This broken promise has resulted in the pluralistic health care environment that we have explored, with community members forced to navigate among ever-changing options based on what is available and what they can afford. As a result, effective treatment has come to be conflated with cost, and health is viewed as a commodity. Poor Maya residents of Chimaltenango recognize all too clearly that the wealthy have access to superior, private health care—that wealth equals health. Well-off parents can buy expensive ORT products for their children, like bottled solutions and Omnilife products.

Waning global health efforts on ORT underscore for poor mothers that they are on their own.

Global health campaigns contribute to the shifting nature of the pluralistic neoliberal health care landscape as priority areas come and go, and programs are begun but not funded forever. Global health perpetuates relationships of control and indebtedness between donor and recipients, from individuals like Ceci taking what they can from programs to national governments like Guatemala that must accede to the terms of foreign governments and donors. In the push toward sustainability, programs built with foreign aid often become fee-for-service, potentially excluding their intended population in order to financially survive. The need for programs to be self-sustaining without ongoing government or NGO support creates the kind of pluralistic health care marketplace we see in Guatemala—rich with the neoliberal dream of choice and exclusivity for those who can pay. Choice, then, becomes about control.

In considering the relationships of individuals to social institutions, Mary Douglas asserted that "bodily control is an expression of social control."[37] From the early 2000s, Guatemala has had a series of hardline populist presidential administrations. Several recent presidential campaigns have appealed to voters with promises of reining in the high crime rates and corruption of prior administrations through a *mano dura* or "strong hand." Political posters with a fist raised are jarring in the Guatemalan context where *so* much control has always been exerted by the elite. Yet the elite campaign and win elections on the (somehow unironic) premise that all Guatemala needs is *more* of their control for conditions to improve. The Guatemalan health system exerts control over Maya bodies through services forced on them, such as vaccinations, services denied to them, like consistent access to low-cost ORT, and services unavailable to them, like costly private clinics. The distribution of health care resources is another way of maintaining the existing strict social hierarchy, primarily through the increase of imbalanced power relations that are introduced through biomedicine.[38] Yet the body politic of poor, Indigenous communities does not passively submit to control and regulation imposed by the health system. Individuals and communities push back against perceived limitations on their autonomy and refuse at times to submit to the care of government health workers.[39] Nongovernment options, even costly and unattainable ones, can feel like freedom of choice.

Global Health Funding Limitations

Choice and control in global health are also shaped by metrics. The impact of ORT campaigns has been evaluated primarily in terms of child mortality and morbidity. And, as explored in chapter 1, it has been a transformative global health success! Government programs depend on metrics to show fidelity to program plans as well as impact, maximizing opportunities for political capital and continuing infusions of economic capital. NGOs, forged in the same neoliberal fire as government programs, face an existential need for results, justifying their work and continued need to donors. In fact, data-driven notions of altruism hold that we can and should apply rationality to philanthropy to consider how our resources can make the greatest impact.[40] But just as external actors set global health, development, and humanitarian agendas, they also set the agenda for measuring impact and determining success. Metrics obscure the lived experiences of recipients of global health programs and who they may have excluded. They can hide hard truths about how effective global health strategies are. For example, Guatemala surpassed its Millennium Development Goals target for improved water supply, reaching 91 percent of the population with access.[41] However, many rural communities received more piped water, but that water has not been not reliably treated. Women in Panaj proudly showed me their new spigots but then, in seemingly unrelated conversation, discussed how their children were having more diarrhea. The metrics on big successes can hide remaining challenges in working toward global health equity.

Sometimes it feels like global health funding cannot win. If it supported ongoing health systems operation in majority world countries, it would only perpetuate the clientelism that continues to plague our global political economy. Yet, when funding creates priory areas, implements programs, and then puts the onus of sustainability on overburdened national governments, programs fizzle. There is so much discussion of health systems strengthening as part of working toward universal health coverage and how weak governance—unsupportive laws, poor management systems, and corruption—is a key barrier.[42] But the imbalanced power dynamics of our global capitalist economy (and the colonial structures on which it is built) created the conditions for which populations of the global majority are then blamed. We must address the structures that create and perpetuate the multivalent violence of inequity in global health.

Global Health Perpetuating Structural Violence: Empowerment and Other Illusions of Equity

Global health is overlaid on colonial structures, and it—however unwittingly—replicates those inherently unequal structures as it strives for global health equity. Well-intentioned infusions of goods and services can worsen inequalities within a recipient country rather than improve them. On this point, Michael Marmot states, "Relief of such material deprivation is not simply a technical matter of providing clean water or better medical care. Who gets these resources is socially determined."[43] Foreign aid can cause harm by funding the very political and economic systems that perpetuate structural violence. Beyond the financial strings that tie majority world nations to high-income country indebtedness, the processes of global health implementation further maintain the status quo. Technical expertise in global health evokes the cycle of resource extraction from the majority world during colonization; it is built on the raw materials taken from the colonized and given value once in the territory of the colonizer. The epidemiologic data collected by local community health workers and mobile health teams are harvested and passed up the global health food chain to high-income countries, where they are used by "experts" to make policy decisions, plan programs, and train students (ensuring a continuing supply of experts). The expertise of local workers and health system leaders is undervalued, and their experiences of actually doing the work of global health through program implementation too often gets lost in the process of data analysis, program evaluation, and economic valuation.

Global health and development strategies are created by experts who are often distant from the lived experiences of the programs they create and the populations they seek to help. The pooling of scientific knowledge and implementation best practices creates essential resources for majority world countries. The WHO provides the gold standard of global health clinical guidelines: furnishing relevant scientific information, epidemiologic data, biomedical best practices, and intervention toolkits (which include materials for training staff); establishing supply and information systems; and implementing and evaluating programs. WHO guidelines are developed from evidence-based knowledge and practice by drawing together advisory panels of topical experts from across the globe, increasingly working toward balancing the hegemony of high-income country experts with those from majority world contexts. WHO toolkits are then developed to make the guidance as straightforward as possible for health systems leaders to implement. These tookits are vital to global health equity because they provide detailed guidance that many countries do not have the technical capacity to develop on their own guidelines. The global guidelines shared in toolkits always emphasize the importance of adapting to local cultures and conditions. This is critical to program success, but it is often given short shrift. As we have seen in the case of ORT in Guatemala, one size programming does not fit all, and it enables the structural violence that maintains the societal status quo.

The Violence of Racialized Health Delivery

In Guatemala, national development programs have largely viewed the Indigenous population as primitive and, thus, as cultural and racial barriers to progress, modernity, and development. Internal development efforts have focused on the assimilation of the Mayan population into mainstream Guatemalan culture and lifestyles.[44] This is a pattern repeated across Latin America, as recently adopted constitutions and treaties may pay lip service to goals of creating multicultural societies but inequalities in power structures remain.[45] Among government ministries working toward development goals, there is little cooperation and communication on the ground. Paul Farmer used structural violence to refer to social structures that "put people in harm's way."[46] The Guatemalan Ministry of Health is ill-equipped to address entrenched ethnic inequalities in access to health care, and its budget and political pull are weak in comparison to other branches of government. The poorly funded Guatemalan government health system continues to put people in harm's way.

One afternoon when I was still a graduate student, I tagged along with a Ministry of Health colleague to a meeting convened by a multilateral government organization in Guatemala City to discuss intermediate progress on a child nutritional supplementation program. I sat in a row of chairs behind the huge wooden conference table and listened. The foreign coordinator reminded everyone of the program's objectives and the responsibilities that each team member had. Then, in turn, each regional implementation manager reported on how much powdered nutritional supplement their area had distributed and the aggregate growth metrics of children in their region. After each man (they were all men, mostly *ladino*) had spoken, the foreign coordinator sighed and dropped his head into his hands. "Why aren't we seeing any changes? Any improvements?" he asked. Everyone murmured and ventured guesses about needing more time, although the program had been running for more than a year. As suggestions petered out, I realized my hand was raised. The foreign coordinator tipped his head questioningly. I then told the group that maybe I could help explain because I was currently living in a rural village that was part of the intervention. I told them that people in the community wanted what was best for their kids and wanted them to grow. But they did not give the nutritional supplement to their kids. They fed it to their chickens. The room exploded with exclamations and comments about the futility of doing any interventions among "the Maya." When things settled down a bit, I explained that the nutritional supplement was being distributed in bags that looked like animal feed, so people fed it to their chickens. No one would give their kids animal feed! But community members were happy that their chickens laid more eggs, which they could eat or sell in the market. The program had benefits, even nutritional ones, just not through the pathway they intended.

This story again illustrates how much aggregate numbers from global health interventions can hide, but it also shows the thoughtful agency of community members. They are not empty vessels just sitting around waiting on someone to come and tell them how to live.[47] In fact, they are alternately bemused and confused (and sometimes angered) by the strange programs that wind their way down the mountain roads into their communities. Global health campaigns are often paternalistic in their assumption that they know what is best for the targeted population. A blame the victim attitude prevails, as Nurit Guttman and William Harris Ressler articulate: "By saying that people need to be responsible for their health behaviors, we imply that they are culpable for adverse consequences when they do not adopt preventive measures."[48] Therefore, community members become liable for the "success" or "failure" of ORT and other global health programs because it is supposedly their responsibility to adopt the advocated practice.[49] Within ORT campaigns in Guatemala, in a particular case of an oft-repeated global phenomenon, the assumptions of global health programs are patterned by racism and gender bias.

Programs, developed in Geneva, Atlanta, or other global health metropoles and implemented by centralized government authorities and their partners, diminish community autonomy because they disallow meaningful community input. For example, we need only to remember the vaccination drive in Guatemala when mobile health teams jokingly threatened rural Maya populations that the police would lock them up if they did not come out for vaccination. While this incident may have been funny to the educated, urban health team members, the rural population that had been the target of massacres by soldiers and police years earlier was not amused. This did lasting harm to community engagement with health services. Beyond the obvious racism, we can also see that government health programs are implemented in a coercive way, rather than as a participatory, shared social good.

Another way community autonomy is diminished is through the definition of who constitutes a "community."[50] Communities on the maps of the walls of Guatemalan health centers do not map onto local people's affinities and understanding of their community. For example, Rosario was "assigned" to the health post at Simejuleu, but she and many others in Panaj had relatives in a larger village with a health post just a bit further in the opposite direction. Communities do not fit neatly into health system catchment areas. This misrecognition, the symbolic violence of imposing community, carves people into groups by geography or ethnicity or language, enabling differential treatment as though it is the natural order.

Further, too often community participation or stakeholder engagement are little more than fashionable global health buzzwords and do not result in meaningful relationship-building.[51] Rather, they become quick efforts to get communities to agree to whatever was already planned. Though couched in terms of empowerment, the community participation element of health interventions often refers to cultural translation of a centralized program or global toolkit to "make it work" in community settings. Rarely do these programs solicit input about the most important health issues a community faces from their own perspective.[52] Maya peoples in Chimaltenango are expected to be passive recipients of health education and services and do not have input on how ORT or other interventions are designed and implemented. The one-way nature of health programming is more marked among rural populations, where community members are expected to be both grateful recipients and active participants in whatever shows up on a truck.

Women as Handmaidens of Equity and Empowerment

The passivity expected of Maya communities in global health delivery is redoubled through global health programs focused on women. Often framed as empowerment, women are made the targets of global health programs under the assumption that they will be the primary caregivers of their children, paradoxically burdening them with responsibility for the success of the program. Mothers are asked by diarrhea prevention education programs to change their daily habits of cooking, cleaning, and childcare, and then to take on the labor of giving ORT when a child has diarrhea. ORT recommendations can go against social and familial norms and may require resources not available within the household, but then women are blamed for poor outcomes if they have not followed the recommendations. They are dammed if they do, dammed if they don't. For example, women in the village of Panaj have repeatedly been told to boil their drinking water, but very few of them do because gathering firewood is time-consuming or costly if purchased. If a child gets diarrhea, fault-finding neighbors might ask if the mother boiled the water. When diarrhea occurs, mothers typically make choices and use their own money for local treatments, including community health workers, traditional healers, and pharmacies; yet, their husbands decide to initiate major treatment-seeking, like a trip to health facility.

Although global health education programs center on women, intending to 'empower' them with knowledge and choices, they, in turn, have the task of convincing their husbands that a particular choice is necessary. While most women are the decision-makers when it comes to seeking low-cost, local treatments, this is not always the case. For example, in chapter 3, we met Juana in Panaj, whose husband forced her to hide from the mobile health teams. Because of her husband's fear of interacting with the government, Juana's choices in seeking health care for her children were severely limited. Women's unpaid labor is a bedrock of global health programming on two fronts, through: 1) participation and action expected of community members; 2) accepting roles as community health workers and other low-level, frontline health workers to do the hard work of program implementation in communities. Women, who already contribute vast amounts of unpaid labor to their families and society, are expected to do still more for global health. Women's unpaid labor does not align with the values of empowerment and equity that global health means to advance, and this issue is finally beginning to receive increased attention and critique within global health.[53]

Cultural Violence and Autonomy

Just as many Maya community members shy away from government health services because of the history of the internal armed conflict and continuing exclusion, development efforts to increase social participation in community decision-making have been challenging, with pronounced power asymmetries between community members and institutional and government representatives.[54] Advocacy networks can be built, but they ultimately may not be guided by—or even participated in—by those for whom they are intended to advocate. The information politics of advocacy networks have a life of their own. After sustained NGO efforts focusing on human rights education in Guatemala over the past twenty years, it is now common, in my observation, for rural Maya women to use human rights terminology in discussing their situation and their goals. It is less common, however, for them to be in leadership roles of the NGOs that advocate for their rights and teach empowerment.

In Guatemala, cultural violence rooted in the othering of Maya populations retrenches racist and classist ideologies and control of resources. Cultural violence refers to the use of aspects of culture to justify or legitimize direct or structural violence.[55] Health services and other social goods are distributed on the terms of the powerful—proximally the ruling elite and the government agencies they control and distally the high-income country experts and leaders. Many times over the years I have heard limited expansions of health services in Maya communities justified because "they" have their own beliefs, "they" do not want health care. Such cultural violence is abetted by global health toolkits that encourage homogenized approaches to health problems with complex local realities.

The result is poor health outcomes for poor Maya populations. The failures of affordable, available, accessible, quality health care—the cornerstones for the delivery of health as a human right—are obscured, hidden in the underbelly of global health program evaluation and outcome metrics. Then, poor outcome metrics are used as a reason to doubt more resources will help. The emphasis is on getting the Maya to make the "right" choices rather than on program planners to anticipate challenges or solicit meaningful input from communities. This is the unfair burden put on marginalized, racialized, and excluded communities across the globe. The powerful want the choices that individuals in these groups make—choices constrained by every global-to-local tier of their marginalization—to align with their own decisions and vested interests. When they cannot or do not, poor health outcomes are implicitly understood to be the result of not being appropriately rational actors within the neoliberal political economy.

Development Burnout and the Hidden Consequences of Global Health

During my very first week in Guatemala, a foreign global health worker said, "The only good thing about Guatemala is it doesn't have suicide bombers." I thought, "Yikes, you need to go home!" While I was disgusted by the way she expressed it at the time, I can now understand her frustration. While challenges faced by global health and development workers in Guatemala are variations on themes played out around the globe, the influx of aid to Guatemala has left aid-targeted people and communities apathetic and wary of new programming. Particularly since the Peace Accords of 1996, Guatemala has experienced a huge boom in development projects and foreign-initiated NGOs. Innumerable NGOs now work in the country; volunteer tourism, where short-term visitors can sign on to help with health, construction, and education projects, is increasingly popular. Yet these projects have little to no oversight and no coordination by any government or other regulatory body. Aid recipients, both organizations and individuals, are in a position where they worry that questioning foreign donors or complaining will result in the loss of that aid. Guatemalans are left feeling they should just take whatever they can get from aid organizations and not have high expectations for the longevity of any one project.

Several years ago, I was trying to convince a senior colleague at global health NGO Partners in Health to expand programming in Guatemala. I thought I was making progress with my pitch, but then he said that Partners in Health could not in good conscience dedicate more of its limited funds toward increased involvement in Guatemala. He talked about how the corruption of the Guatemalan government and the failure to improve the rural infrastructure, despite substantial inputs from multilateral international aid organizations, the US government, and numerous NGOs, indicate that further funding would not be put to good use. He said, "Guatemala is a development dump, and everyone knows it. Aid just seems to disappear there, and nothing really changes."

On the receiving end, having so many different groups at work on so many different development projects makes it difficult for individuals to know who to trust and how to navigate the shifting options and choose among them. As the quote at the beginning of this chapter eloquently indicates, apathy toward development projects is not just found in aid workers but in recipients as well. Residents of Chimaltenango are rightfully suspicious of new development projects; they wonder why new programs are started when old ones were left to languish and fade away. A justified local strategy is to focus on short-term participation for short-term gains, often in the form of material goods, rather than anticipating long-term involvement by any one project within the community. There have been too many disappointments to expect anything other than more disappointment.

ORT and the Development Machine

It would be an understatement to say that excitement about ORT in Chimaltenango has waned. Multiple programs have come and gone, and more have gone than come in recent years. What has been left behind are confusing messages on how to best purify water within the household and how best to make and administer ORT. The government continues to provide ORT packets and give mothers instructions on how to mix them with water and give them to children, along with intermittent water, sanitation, and hygiene educational programs. Various NGOs have also worked in ORT and diarrhea prevention programming, but there are currently no active programs dedicated to systematic ORT education. The vacuum caused by the lack of thorough ORT training has in part been filled by expensive products from pharmacies and companies such as Omnilife that cannot be expected to provide comprehensive ORT education at the point of sale.

There have been insufficient infrastructural changes in Guatemala to make ORT superfluous: the water supply and living conditions of the poor, in both urban and rural settings, continue to be a significant source of diarrheal pathogens. In fact, 88 percent of all cases of diarrhea in the majority world are attributable to poor water, sanitation, and hygiene; these findings are echoed by a Guatemalan study.[56] In Guatemala, a staggering 98 percent of water sources are contaminated with *E. coli*.[57] Prevention of diarrheal disease is such a constant, overwhelming task that it often gets ignored as futile. Moreover, ORT is hardly a flashy new global health tool, and ORT interventions are unlikely to produce the immediate, measurable results favored by current public health and development schemes, such as the Sustainable Development Goals. With limited funding and seemingly limitless need, it makes sense to expect programs to produce results and become self-sustaining, but these ideals cannot be reached merely by paying lip service to them.

My conversations with program officials at PAHO and UNICEF Guatemala have highlighted an emphasis on in-country self-sufficiency and attempts to wean programs off international aid packages. In discussing ORT programming, both organizations reported proudly that their role in ORT and largely all primary health care issues has solely become an advisory one and that they no longer actively provide ORT program assistance. The UNICEF official told me that Guatemalan production of oral rehydration salts (ORS) packets is sufficient to meet the requirements of the government health system and its pharmacies, and UNICEF keeps a stockpile of 200,000 ORS packets as part of its emergency preparedness package. However, my research in Chimaltenango has shown that government pharmacies and mobile health teams are often out of ORS packets, indicating that even if enough packets are produced, serious distribution problems remain.

Self-sufficiency and sustainable development models are viewed as unassailable in contemporary aid, global health, and development sectors, as if a fashion for hands-off independence can undo centuries of manipulation and forced dependency. The zeal to achieve sustainability goals, including for ORT programming, has led to a hands-off attitude from multilateral agencies and international NGOs that harms the populations they have spent years and millions of dollars ostensibly assisting. Gains made by previous ORT efforts by the government health system and NGOs are being lost because continued education and ORS packets are not adequately available. Long-term efforts are needed to sustain changes implemented by a global health campaign, and community input is essential for building trust in public programming and creating access to social goods in Guatemala.[58]

ORT should no longer be a necessary public health intervention on a widespread scale in Guatemala or anywhere. Indeed, ORT interventions were conceptualized as a stopgap measure on the road to development, and they would no longer be needed if the world's poor had access to clean water and safe sanitation systems.[59] The Guatemalan government has not provided these social goods for its people, and it also does not allocate adequate resources to the health system to allow for ongoing comprehensive ORT education and distribution. Of course not. Corruption and weak tax structure lead to anemic investment in durable infrastructure and health system strengthening. Everyone, from Maya community members to national advocates to the leadership of global organizations, knows this. Somehow the sum of our global health, development, and human rights parts add up to less than the whole that a just and equitable society require.

Uncoordinated Efforts toward Unclear Progress

The case of global health and development in Guatemala illustrates that too much can mean too little: too many uncoordinated development projects lead to unsatisfactory overall improvements in national development indicators and in people's lives. A fragmented development scheme where projects work in isolation perpetuates structural violence at micro and macro levels. Wealthy *ladinos* in Guatemala, like populations of socioeconomic means anywhere in the world, are not expected to be grateful for crumbs of health care dropped off at random in their communities. They certainly do not tramp miles over steep terrain to find that the health post is out of ORS packets. Yet, these inequalities can be obscured by a surfeit of uncoordinated global health and development projects.

Development projects feed multivalent political and economic interests, often even as they aim to do otherwise.[60] Well-meaning NGOs can exacerbate existing tensions and infuse attention and funds to programs and priorities that go awry in local context.[61] However, just as individuals are agentive in their engagement with global health and development programming, so, too, are low- and middle-income countries in their engagement with the global health and development agendas. They agentively shape their narratives and remake their self-images to maximize investment by the global health and development organizations that framed those particular images and narratives as meritorious of funding.[62] But in doing so, the power of high-income countries and the institutions they control remains unchecked and the global systems of inequality unchanged. There are very few counterexamples to this dynamic; Rwanda is prominent among them in its rejection of foreign aid that does not align with central government strategic goals.[63] However, this exception, in its extreme notability, proves the rule of needy stasis created by our systems of foreign aid.

Current, uncoordinated development efforts cannot begin to address the entrenched racism and discrimination that weight political and economic structures against rural, poor, and Indigenous populations in Guatemala. Maya communities are blamed for holding Guatemala back from "development," as though they are responsible for their own marginalized status, as though they do not desire the social goods that the wealthy enjoy. Global health and development programs continue to pour in funding, but enthusiasm for these gains is leavened with low expectations that real changes in health metrics, much less health equity, will result. As one clear-eyed mother in a village near Acatenango put it, "If we had money to make changes, we would have a clinic with a doctor to attend children with diarrhea. If we had money, we would already have a health center. Someday these changes will come, and we will all live better for it."

So What? Pressure Points for Action in Global Health

There is so much that is broken in our global health systems, and we will not repair them by doing more of the same.[64] More is not working. We must look to the leadership of global health and development experts from the majority world to shape our efforts anew. Simply documenting cultural and structural violence does not build health equity, but thoughtful action guided by the communities who experience these persistent forms of violence can. Social suffering demands social action. Global health must finally be a truly global project—we collectively have a moral and ethical obligation to dismantle the systems of inequality established by conquest and colonization that continue to flourish under neoliberalism. I believe we can excise the underbelly.

So much important work is happening to explore decolonizing global health. From the way that researchers from high-income countries generate and publish data to the way that global health education is structured and delivered, there are clear and actionable steps we can take.[65] Decolonizing global health is necessarily a multitiered mandate, from individuals to organizations to our systems and superstructures.[66] And there is so much that gives me hope that we can meaningfully build a decolonial global health and make strides toward health equity in Guatemala and beyond. For example, at the global level, the Brocher Declaration calls for building equitable global health partnerships, with a focus on holding short-term global health travel experiences accountable for their operational ethics and mindfulness of the power differentials between visiting teams of foreign volunteers and local recipient communities.[67] Good intentions can be made better! At the national level in Guatemala, efforts like EcoFiltro, a social enterprise dedicated to provision of clean water to the poor through household water filters, builds a bridge between the exclusionary impacts of privatization and the failures of government to build durable water, sanitation, and hygiene infrastructure.[68] Finally, at the local level, Guatemalan groups like the Maya Health Alliance, the Population Council Guatemala, Women's Justice Institute, and Center for the Study of Equity and Governance in Health Systems do the slow and steady work of building community consensus on priorities, gender equity, and engagement in health and development programming.[69]

Our systems-level focus in global health can lead us to forget that individuals and communities are not passive recipients of health and development programs. We must foreground the rationale, priorities, and preferences of communities, particularly among populations like Maya peoples in Guatemalan who have faced repression and control of historic proportions, in how we shape global health programs. We can work to dismantle the truism that health equals wealth by building systems that support the human right to health, but we must recognize that these systems will not be framed in a WHO toolkit or outlined in an international conference presentation. They will be created by the people for whom they will work—global health actors, structures, and systems just have to listen.

Conclusion

This book has introduced health in the particular worlds of highland Guatemala and Maya communities, but its stories are echoed in marginalized communities across the majority world. Childhood diarrheal disease continues to cause lasting developmental consequences and death in Guatemala, a mundane reality unimaginable in high-income countries. Childhood diarrhea can typically be managed through home use of oral rehydration therapy (ORT), first developed to manage cholera outbreaks where demand for intravenous fluids outstripped availability. ORT has become a ubiquitous part of the global health community education and programming landscape, and it has saved about 70 million young lives over the past fifty years.[1] The successes of ORT have been rarely matched in global health—it is a technologically simple solution requiring no specialized supply chains and, in fact, can be made with ingredients found in even the most resource-constrained homes. However, the metrics of success obscure the underbelly of global health—the reality that our programs reinscribe patterns of inequality both globally and locally.

ORT has mainly been understood within global health as an effort in knowledge transfer and behavior change. However, its successes are patterned by social inequalities, like all social goods. The preference from global health organizations for manufactured solutions and the scientific specificity of their formula has had far-reaching effects. In particular, the relatively labor-intensive work of administering ORT falls to women who are almost exclusively the targets of childhood diarrhea interventions in global health. These educational efforts, often delivered with instructions at odds with the infrastructure and material reality of women's lives, are framed as empowering women. But women are blamed for failures to implement the water, sanitation, and hygiene messages typically coupled with ORT education. The penetration of diarrhea prevention and treatment messages is deep enough that stigma surrounds mothers whose children experience diarrhea, but the infrastructure—despite great successes on the Millennium Development Goals—has not removed the ever-present threat of childhood diarrhea. Women, then, are doubly burdened by the patriarchal norms of Guatemalan society and by the expectations of global health programs that seek to empower them.

Although ORT has been widely promoted over the past fifty years, many people in highland Guatemala do not realize that they can create their own oral rehydration solution from materials in their home, and they buy into the idea that better treatments cost more money. Within a government health system designed to exclude them, many Maya people are wary of seeking health care from government services and often face difficulties in accessing the scant services available because of distance, ancillary costs, and racism. These barriers make private options particularly appealing, and the neoliberal Guatemalan health care landscape offers a riot of options—from traditional healers to drug sellers and pharmacies to nongovernmental organizations (NGOs) and private clinics to short-term medical missions. Although the pluralistic health care environment seems to offer freedom of choice, it ensnares care-seekers in a web of complex choices in which money (and other forms of capital) is the final arbiter.

In fact, the pluralistic health care system in Guatemala is less a system and more a confusion. Health care offerings come and go, compounded by development dumping by foreign organizations beginning in the post–civil war era of the mid-1990s. Well-intended programs, campaigns, and interventions funded by foreign governments and NGOs clash with both Guatemalan government priorities and with each other. Too much (money, programs, effort) has meant too little (sustained improvement, health systems strengthening). Too many development efforts have also led to development burnout in which everyone involved—global health and development workforces, government implementation teams, and community members—feels a sense of futility and knows that the current effort will be gone in the next budget cycle. ORT programs represent a microcosm of global health writ large, where global guidelines misalign with local realities but the power dynamics of funding and the distant authority of experts insist that things be done a certain way. Those same power dynamics then cascade locally, following well-worn channels of in-country inequalities. By the time a global health campaign on ORT (or anything else) reaches local communities, it has been shaped by every tier of the global political economy except their own.

The Underbelly of This Book—the (Un)necessary Anthropologist

I showed up in Guatemala in 2005 with a list of organizations working on childhood diarrhea and ORT. I was delighted when a local health organization wanted to partner on the research that I hoped to do on diarrhea; we agreed to collaborate, and I promised to return with grant funding. When I walked back into the director's office nearly a year later, he laughed until he cried, saying they never thought they would see me again. It was my first lesson on how global health on the ground can be full of empty promises. I grew up in the 1990s, a part of the Model UN generation and a time when well-intentioned (if deeply flawed) multiculturalism taught us that greater global cooperation and equity were within our grasp. We were led to believe that progress toward the unequivocal good of human rights and social justice, however difficult, was unidirectional and inevitable. However naive an American high schooler pretending to be on the UN Human Rights Council at the turn of the millennium now seems, I still believe in the hopeful conceit of human rights. But I have seen firsthand that they are paper promises and empty words when not backed by sustained collective action.

I have worked as a medical anthropologist in global health and in Guatemala for more than fifteen years now. When I first arrived in Guatemala, my mental map was as flat as an atlas, but it is now populated with friends and memories—the place where I did my first interview in Kaqchikel, the place where friends till the soil for maize to eat and cash crops to sell, the place we celebrated my eldest son's first birthday with a piñata, the place we hosted my goddaughter's quinceañera. There are so many beautiful and challenging places. I continue to interrogate my internal map and the stories that I tell of Guatemala. The ethnographer can only tell the stories that we see and that we live. Our secondhand telling can never capture the reality of the lives of our interlocutors. I have struggled to know which stories should be told and which should be held close, the weight of them multiplying over the years.

So now I must tell you the underbelly of this book. Throughout its pages, I deeply feel the absence of a friend and colleague who was murdered during our shared work to support community organizing and health projects. My brilliant Maya friend was targeted, tortured, and killed because his work challenged the status quo of power and wealth that has shackled his people for five centuries now. When my friend died—when his broken body was left in a muddy ditch, found too late for the kind of salvation medicine can provide—I wanted justice. Honestly, in my despair, I wanted the kind of justice that would feel like vengeance. I wanted the perpetrators to pay for taking this bright Maya leader from his family, from his community, and from our discussions of social justice by the kitchen fire. I wanted for him to be able to tell you the stories of his community in these pages. In the end, what his family and I wanted did not matter. When the cold light of dawn breaks over a broken body, it illuminates the stark reality that human rights are not for everyone—they are not even safe for everyone to pursue. As the specter of a trial and the resulting publicity became real for his family, it became clear that the clunky mechanisms for making universal human rights a reality could not map onto the local community where my slain friend's mother passes by the perpetrators on her way to the weekly market.[2] This catastrophe has shaped a family. It has shaped a Maya community in highland Guatemala and circumscribed limits on the imaginations of its people for building a more equitable society. And it has shaped my own approach to global health and community-centered work.[3]

I am honored to share pieces of the lives and stories of friends and community members in Guatemala that they have agreed to share, but I cannot and will not speak for others. Maya communities have their own strong voices. I can listen. The ethnographic role of sitting still, of being, of absorbing all that is around us can feel anathema to the global health ethos of working toward social justice and health for all. The privilege of my position as a global health scholar-practitioner from a high-income country means that I can sometimes facilitate resources not readily accessible to local communities. However, anthropologists, development workers, global health program officers, and our kin are not *necessary* to local communities. We too often serve as the flimsiest of bandages on the wounds wrought by the systems of inequality that seem to grow only deeper through our neoliberal political economy. We can work to change the taken-for-granted dynamic of "locals" and "foreign" aid experts—global health must center marginalized communities in the global majority world to move toward social justice and the achievement of health as a human right.

Co-design for Global Health

The weight of centuries of global power dynamics and inequality can seem insurmountable as global health works toward decolonization—an endeavor worth every inch gained, even while the goal remains elusive. Our field must do everything we can to be accountable for our past and work toward a different future. Global health has been critiqued as "old wine in new bottles," as a rebranding of international health and the tropical hygiene and colonial medicine eras that came before.[4] We can both recognize the historical and continuing forces of inequality at play and also work to dismantle them, however imperfectly. It is time to make something new with the ingredients of global health—time to make sangria with that old wine.

Within discussions of decolonizing global health, there are many important analyses of the global political economy of health and development funding—the macrostructures of global health. There are also many vital and actionable discussions of how high-income country experts and organizations can work more fairly—the micro-interactions of global health in the field. However, I am concerned there is a gap between the micro and macro that is under-addressed in efforts to decolonize global health. What are the program paradigms and approaches that will enable us to meaningfully reorient our work toward equitable processes that yield equitable outcomes in global health? Co-design is one approach that provides an opportunity to balance the resources of global health and development, through pooled expertise and funding, with local needs and priorities.

Over my years of working in Guatemala, observing many global health and development failures, including my own, I can see that only projects defined by and shaped by communities are successful. Co-design has the potential to be a transformative paradigm shift in global health.[5] Co-design, both a philosophy and a process, recognizes that the health care landscape reflects social norms and intentionally works to remake that landscape by focusing on community-identified needs. The philosophy is of radical decentering of traditional expertise during program design in order to center community collaboration. This can help rebalance power both in decision-making and in the allocation of resources.

The co-design process that I work with merges components of agile design thinking, rapid ethnography, and public health intervention mapping. A team, led by community partners, works through six steps in an iterative process. First, priority community needs and project goals are established with the community. Second, we collectively conduct a needs assessment and asset analysis, recognizing that there are existing strengths and resources. Third, we explore existing solutions and possible innovations to build upon. Fourth, we refine a prototype of the co-designed innovation; sometimes it is a new technology, but it can also be an adapted program design or novel delivery technique. Several cycles of steps three and four help optimize the innovation and incorporate input from groups beyond the co-design team. Fifth, end-users are trained on the co-designed innovation. Sixth, the innovation is implemented, and ongoing evaluation allow continuous improvement and refining. Co-design is both human-centered and agile, meaning that design processes prioritize rapid cycles of innovation, trial, and revision. Co-design, by its nature, is flexible and human-centered—qualities that global health programs often lack.

Co-design centers communities in the work of global health, creating a structure for meaningful community engagement.[6] Superficial cultural adaptation or a few stakeholder engagement meetings are not enough, but co-design can be a real method for prioritizing people's needs rather than imposing solutions.[7] Yet, it risks the pitfalls of all global health trends by becoming a buzzword we say and not a process we do. There is a rapidly growing literature describing co-designed projects in global health, but most do not describe their processes in any detail, which limits our ability to learn and build best practices.[8]

Co-design is also not devoid of power dynamics; it requires ongoing reflexivity and questioning of power dynamics and renegotiation of roles to maintain equitable codesign partnerships.[9] There are no quick fixes for achieving social justice or health system strengthening. Co-design takes investment of time and resources. Because co-designed projects do not have a priori outcomes, they do not necessarily neatly slot into global metrics. The co-design approach creates heterogeneous programs and data, but it can make each project count. Co-design can ensure programs are identified, desired, and shaped by the communities where they are implemented. While global health can draw on shared knowledge and lessons learned, we will never achieve universal health coverage or the universal human right to health with universal approaches.

Remaking Global Health

The arc of change will not bend toward social justice unless its light is refracted by stakeholders working to dismantle the unjust power dynamics of contemporary global health and development. The prism of global health is held by the political and economic elites of high-income countries and, to some degree, by people like me, well-meaning experts from those same countries. We must invert the prism to center local needs and desires. The metropoles of global health must shift from the likes of Geneva, London, Boston, and Atlanta to Lagos, New Delhi, and Guatemala City. These points of confluence in the majority world have the expertise and leadership to do the work of a new, decolonial global health, and they must be funded accordingly.[10] This essential decentering of high-income countries and their spheres of influence will not achieve global health equity alone. We must also acknowledge in funding mechanisms and implementation models that the benefits of foreign global health and development aid are too often distributed inequitably within countries, as the example of Guatemala has so starkly illustrated.

We must repopulate our map of global health actors and power brokers. The decolonization of global health will not be led by high-income country experts like me but by the experts in communities everywhere.[11] We can all play a role in improving global health, but we must prioritize the expertise and stories of the majority world. The human right to health should not be a whim of geography or constrained by the contents of wallets. Fundamentally, the attainment of the right to health does not rest on individual choices—an illusory freedom in an unfair marketplace made mandatory by neoliberalism—but on systems that create high-quality options for everyone. Co-design is one tool that can help build global health equity and dissolve the underbelly of global health.

Afterword

Arthur Kleinman

Underbelly is an important book. Like other medical anthropology studies, it offers a powerful critique of local, national, and global social conditions that come together to cause disease and block effective health interventions, especially among the poor. Yet, Rachel Hall-Clifford goes beyond critique in order to show how the co-design approach to health interventions with local families and communities can establish the favorable conditions that support durable outcomes. In this particular instance, we see how poor, rural Guatemalan families respond to their children's repeated experiences of diarrheal disease and how that could be improved.

Here the ethnographer becomes an intervener. Hall-Clifford's approach to intervention is to work with local mothers and communities to create the conditions for oral rehydration therapy (ORT) and other social technologies to become safe and feasible to treat children suffering from repeated diarrhea. Thereby the cycle of "diarrhea, dehydration, health complications, death" can be broken and children can survive, while families gain the mastery of key treatments and the confidence to use them.

Underbelly canvasses all the major issues facing global health today: social suffering and structural violence; social and health inequalities; racism; colonialism; profound poverty; institutional failures in NGO governance and performance; and more. But rather than leave the reader feeling frustrated if not hopeless, Hall-Clifford follows the path built by Paul Farmer and Partners in Health by raising the voices of marginal families and communities as she works toward a more optimistic and promising future for her protagonists. As Farmer emphasized, the problems we face in global health result from treating others as if they count for less. Hall-Clifford's moral imagination transcends this existential evil. No one counts for less in this challenging yet uplifting book.

Heretofore, much of global health research has focused on the admittedly more basic question of improving access to health services. Now the question that should be asked is, *What is the quality of such services?* And not simply those services offered by professionals but those deployed by families and communities. My own impression after a half century of witnessing global health caregiving is that the quality is often lower than what we anticipate, or rather hope for, and in reality is hardly ever measured. There are two reasons for this failure to measure the quality of care. To begin with, we still lack routine measures of quality of care, particularly outside of health facilities. And we are all-too-often willing to accept, just as virtually all health care systems today do, the substitution of measures of institutional efficiency as surrogates for quality. Of course, they are not and can never be.

Quality should be exactly what Hall-Clifford herself demonstrates in her warm, respectful, and supportive relationships with her interlocutors: person-centered and socially responsive to local life. Quality care includes (1) establishing a respectful therapeutic relationship based on reciprocity; (2) the animated presence of practitioners and patients and family members; (3) adequate time spent together; (4) interview skills; (5) listening; (6) communicating effectively and responding to questions; and (7) skill in physical examination, appropriate use of laboratories, diagnosis, and treatment. Simply listing these things illustrates how infrequently the impoverished Maya mothers we have encountered in this book experienced anything approaching quality care. We also become aware that quality care and prevention for Hall-Clifford means involvement of families and communities right from the start in developing needs assessment. The perceptions and values of real people and the local worlds in which they live thus become as important as the perceptions and values of global health experts in program development.

Is it then permissible to write off such quality care as something the poor cannot now or perhaps ever experience? The answer should be a resounding no. That answer rejects the socialization-for-scarcity model that has come to dominate global public health. That model insists that the poor cannot receive the same quality of care that other people receive because they lack the resources to pay for it. Poor communities deserve high quality, and it can be delivered with proper training, increased mobilization of already available resources, and support of caregivers, together with serious evaluation of the care they provide. Right now, we do not measure quality of care in global health, and patients do not expect quality care. This is the world as described by Hall-Clifford that needs to change.

What is needed is to reimagine health care systems in such a way that care, not money, becomes a central value. For most of us, this is a difficult thought experiment because we are so accustomed to taking for granted that care is to be purchased as a product and that the consumer-provider model of caregiving is the one we feel we must accept, despite the powerful reservations that many of us harbor. And Hall-Clifford shows that even extremely poor Maya families will pay for private practitioners instead of receiving free government care because it means higher quality—or at least the perception of it. Accompanied by the famous Indian anthropologist Veena Das, I saw several decades ago much the same dynamic in a slum in New Delhi. In that slum, the offices of private practitioners surrounded the informal settlements and alleyways damp with sewage in a predatory setting. Despite the expense of private care, terribly poor people had to pay for treatment; they did so since it was more available and perceived to be better than what was on offer in government clinics. Over the past decades, I have observed much the same situation among poor communities in several Southeast Asian and African countries. Indeed, the conditions for care among the poor in the United States share some of the same features. In the United States, even the middle class is poorly served by a chaotic, broken, and exploitive health care system in which money, not care, is prioritized. In China, where I do my research, a great deal of effort has been made to lift the rural poor out of poverty, and it has met with success. China has poured money into rural development, including health care systems. While real improvements have occurred, some of the same problems described by Hall-Clifford still exist.

Notwithstanding the absence of on-the-ground models, it is our responsibility to reimagine a radically different circumstance of care if we are to witness the development of policies and plans for health systems reform that actually make quality care a reality. To accomplish this, I am convinced that we need to build or rebuild health systems by making care a public good and adequate quality of care the right of the people. The thought experiment accelerates as we come to terms with the fact that whether the economic system is neoliberal capitalism, state capitalism, or socialist capitalism, we all swim in a sea of capitalism. Short of a revolution that changes this reality, and I see no evidence that such is coming, the best that we can do is to organize care as a public good. Neither the marketplace nor a state-controlled public health care system can create the conditions for good care unless we insist that, in fact, is our starting point.

The most revolutionary idea is to imagine a health system today that begins with care as its core value and central practice and then work backward to figure out how to create this as a reality, not in some imagined utopia but in the dust and smoke of real communities. Can Maya villages, for example, be organized in such a way that even with an incomplete and imperfect project of poverty reduction, care systems can be built with available resources to structure care in a more adequate manner? This is why policymakers and program planners should read this ethnography and others like it. Hall-Clifford describes the problems that need to be resolved and the opportunities that need to be enhanced if quality care is to become even a modest reality in the Guatemalan highlands and in others of the poorest communities in the world. What the correct balance should be between local communities, NGOs, the nation-state, private society, and the international order is something that needs to be—and can be—figured out if, and only if, our reimagination of global health delivery begins and ends with the care of real people in real contexts as its core concern.

Underbelly provides the ethnographic reality for this work of reimagination to begin. It is to be hoped that global health experts, at least those with the right values, will take up the challenge and work to answer the question it poses, not just for the Guatemalan highlands but for the very different local worlds of the poor worldwide: What is good care, and how can it be advanced for people in this particular context?

Arthur Kleinman, MD, MA

Professor of Medical Anthropology,
Department of Global Health and Social Medicine

Professor of Psychiatry, School of Medicine

Rabb Professor, Department of Anthropology

Harvard University
Cambridge, Massachusetts USA

Notes

Prologue

1. Quoted in Skylight Pictures. 2011. *Granito: How to Nail a Dictator*. Director, Pamela Yates. Producer, Paco De Onís.

Introduction

1. Pan American Health Organization (PAHO). 2017. *Health in the Americas: Guatemala country report*, accessed March 10, 2022, https://www.paho.org/salud-en-las-americas-2017.

2. Comisión para el Esclarecimiento Histórico (CEH). 1999. *Guatemala, memoria del silencio*. Oficina de Servicios para Proyectos de las Naciones Unidas (UNOPS).

3. Benson, P., and Fisher, E. 2009. Social suffering in Guatemala's postwar era: Mayas in postwar Guatemala. In *Harvest of violence revisited*, 151–166; Little, W. E., & Smith, T. J. (Eds.). University of Alabama Press.; Manz, B. 2008. The continuum of violence in post-war Guatemala. *Social Analysis*, 52(2): 151–164.

4. Famer, P. 2013. Preface. In P. Farmer, J. Y. Kim, A. Kleinman, and M. Basilico (Eds.), *Reimagining global health: An introduction*. Introduction 1–14. University of California Press.

5. Salm, M., Ali, M., Minihane, M., and Conrad, P. 2021. Defining global health: Findings from a systematic review and thematic analysis of the literature. *BMJ Global Health*, 6(6): e005292.

6. Koplan, J. P., Bond, T. C., Merson, M. H., Reddy, K. S., Rodriguez, M. H., Sewankambo, N. K., and Wasserheit, J. N. 2009. Towards a common definition of global health. *The Lancet*, 373(9679): 1993–1995.

7. Khan, T., Abimbola, S., Kyobutungi, C., and Pai, M. 2022. How we classify countries and people—and why it matters. *BMJ Global Health*, 7(6): e009704.

8. When discussing specific economic conditions, I use low- and middle-income country designations from the World Bank where indicated.

9. Packard, R. M. 2016. *A history of global health: Interventions into the lives of other peoples*. Johns Hopkins University Press; Birn, A. E. 2014. Philanthrocapitalism, past and present: The Rockefeller Foundation, the Gates Foundation, and the setting (s) of the international/global health agenda. *Hypothesis*, 12(1): e8; Greene, J., Basilico, M. T., Kim, H., and Farmer, P. 2013. Colonial medicine and its legacies. In P. Farmer, J. Y. Kim, A. Kleinman, and M. Basilico (Eds.), *Reimagining global health: An introduction*, 33–73. University of California Press.

10. Packard, R. M. 2016. *A history of global health: Interventions into the lives of other peoples*. Johns Hopkins University Press.

11. Abimbola, S., Asthana, S., Montenegro, C., Guinto, R. R., Jumbam, D. T., Louskieter, L., Kabubei, K. M., Munshi, S., Muraya, K., Okumu, F., and Saha, S. 2021. Addressing power asymmetries in global health: Imperatives in the wake of the COVID-19 pandemic. *PLoS Medicine*, 18(4): e1003604.

12. Harvey, D. 2007. *A brief history of neoliberalism*. Oxford University Press.

13. Harvey, D. 2007. *A brief history of neoliberalism*. Oxford University Press.

14. Beaudevin, C., Gaudillière, J. P., Gradmann, C., Lovell, A. M., and Pordié, L. 2020. Global health and the new world order: Introduction. In *Global health and the new world order*, 1–28. Manchester University Press.

15. Stapleton, G., Schröder-Bäck, P., Laaser, U., Meershoek, A., and Popa, D. 2014. Global health ethics: An introduction to prominent theories and relevant topics. *Global Health Action*, 7: 23569; Kass, N. E. 2004. Public health ethics: From foundations and frameworks to justice and global public health. *Journal of Law, Medicine & Ethics*, 32: 232–242.

16. Sen, A. 1999. *Development as freedom*. Anchor Books.

17. Million, D. 2013. *Therapeutic nations: Healing in an age of indigenous human rights*. University of Arizona Press.

18. Pratt, B., and Hyder, A. A. 2015. Applying a global justice lens to health systems research ethics: An initial exploration. *Kennedy Institute of Ethics Journal*, 25: 35–66.

19. Fan, E. L. 2021. *Commodities of care: The business of HIV testing in China*. University of Minnesota Press.

20. Adams, V. 2016. *Metrics: What counts in global health*. Duke University Press.

21. Biruk, C. 2018. *Cooking data: Culture and politics in an African research world*. Duke University Press.

22. Biehl, J., and Petryna, A. 2014. Peopling global health. *Saúde e Sociedade*, 23: 376–389.

23. Minn, P. 2022. *Where they need me: Local clinicians and the workings of global health in Haiti*. Cornell University Press.

24. Biehl, J. 2016. Theorizing global health. *Medicine Anthropology Theory*, 3; Carmack, R. M. 1988. *Harvest of violence: The Maya Indians and the Guatemalan crisis*. University of Oklahoma Press.

25. Childress, J. F., Faden, R. R., Gaare, R. D., Gostin, L. O., Kahn, J., Bonnie, R. J., Kass, N. E., Mastroianni, A. C., Moreno, J. D., and Nieburg, P. 2002. Public health ethics: Mapping the terrain. *Journal of Law, Medicine & Ethic*, 30: 170–178; Kass, N. E. 2004. Public health ethics: From foundations and frameworks to justice and global public health. *Journal of Law, Medicine & Ethic*, 32: 232–242.

26. Redfield, P. 2011. The impossible problem of neutrality. In *Forces of compassion: Humanitarianism between ethics and politics*, 53–70. SAR Press; Keshavjee, S. 2014. *Blind spot*. University of California Press; Fassin, D. 2011. *Humanitarian reason: A moral history of the present*. University of California Press; Benatar, S. R. 2013. Global health and justice: Re-examining our values. *Bioethics*, 27: 297–304.

27. Kotsko, A. 2018. *Neoliberalism's demons*. Stanford University Press.

28. Ruger, J. P. 2004. Health and social justice. *The Lancet*, 364(9439): 1075–1080.

29. Bourdieu, P. 2003. *Symbolic violence*. Palgrave Macmillan.

30. The names of some people, places, and identifying details have been changed throughout the book.

31. I could hear the words of Nancy Scheper-Hughes echoing across time as I witnessed the everyday violence of Efraín's suffering and death. Despite my agreement with her ethical analysis of the noninterventionist role of ethnographers (in her incredible *Death without weeping: The violence of everyday life in Brazil*), I confess in the moments of engagement with Rosario and Efraín, I could only care about stopping the suffering in front of me.

32. World Health Organization. 2017. *Diarrhoeal disease*, accessed February 19, 2022, https://www.who.int/news-room/fact-sheets/detail/diarrhoeal-disease. WHO.

33. My husband Gari Clifford is a biomedical engineer who focuses his work on affordable health care technologies for marginalized populations, and we are frequent research collaborators. Any embarrassment about discussion of diarrhea was (fancy) dinner table related!

34. Pan American Health Organization (PAHO). 2017. *Health in the Americas: Guatemala country report*, accessed March 10, 2022, https://www.paho.org/salud-en-las-americas-2017.

35. Maung, K. U., and Greenough, W. B. 1991. Treatment of the dehydrated child. *Pediatric Annals*, 20(1); World Health Organization. 1993. *The management and prevention of diarrhoea: Practical guidelines*. WHO; Cash, R. A. 1983. Oral rehydration

in the treatment of diarrhea: Issues in the implementation of diarrhea treatment programs. In *Diarrhea and malnutrition*, 203–221. Springer; Bentley, M. E., Pelto, G. H., Straus, W. L., Schumann, D. A., Adegbola, C., de la Pena, E., Oni, G. A., Brown, K. H., and Huffman, S. L. 1988. Rapid ethnographic assessment: Applications in a diarrhea management program. Special issue, *Social Science & Medicine*, 27(1): 107–116. https://doi.org/10.1016/0277-9536(88)90168-2; Pebley, A., Hurtado, E., and Goldman, N. 1999. Beliefs about children's illness. *Journal of Biosocial Science*, 31: 195–219.

36. Tedlock, B. 1987. An interpretive solution to the problem of humoral medicine in Latin America. *Social Science & Medicine*, 24: 1069–1083; Hodgkin, C. 1994. North–South network. *Dialogue on Diarrhoea*, 55; Werner, D., Sanders, D., and Weston, J. 1997. *Questioning the solution: The politics of primary health care and child survival, with an in-depth critique of oral rehydration therapy.* HealthWrights. The Millennium Development Goals, established by the United Nations Millennium Declaration in 2000, were eight health and development goals that UN member states agreed to achieve by 2015. They are now followed by the seventeen Sustainable Development Goals target for 2030.

37. Loker, W. M. 1999. Grit in the Prosperity Machine: Globalization and the Rural Poor in Latin America. In W. M. Loker (Ed.), *Globalization and the Rural Poor in Latin America*. Boulder: Lynne Rienner Publishers; Pirttijärvi, J. 1999. *Indigenous Peoples and Development in Latin America*. Ibero-American Center, Univ; PAHO. 2017. *Health in the Americas: Guatemala country report*, accessed March 10, 2022, from https://www.paho.org/salud-en-las-americas-2017.

38. Pan American Health Organization (PAHO). 2017. *Health in the Americas: Guatemala country report*, accessed March 10, 2022, https://www.paho.org/salud-en-las-americas-2017; World Health Organization. 1993. *The management and prevention of diarrhoea: Practical guidelines*. WHO; Gracey, M. 1985. The WHO diarrhoeal diseases control programme. In M. Gracey (Ed.), *Diarrhoeal disease and malnutrition: A clinical update*. 33–54 Churchill Livingstone.

39. Pebley, A., Hurtado, E., and Goldman, N. 1999. Beliefs about children's illness. *Journal of Biosocial Science*, 31: 195–219; Goldman, N., Pebley, A. R., and Gragnolati, M. 2002. Choices about treatment for ARI and diarrhea in rural Guatemala. *Social Science & Medicine*, 55: 1693–1712.

40. Schlesinger, S., and Kinzer, S. 2005. *Bitter fruit: The story of the American coup in Guatemala* (revised and expanded). Harvard University Press.

41. Taylor, C. 2010. *Return of Guatemala's refugees*. Temple University Press.

42. Schlesinger, S., and Kinzer, S. 2005. *Bitter fruit: The story of the American coup in Guatemala* (revised and expanded). Harvard University Press.

43. Taylor, C. 2010. *Return of Guatemala's refugees*. Temple University Press.

44. Menchú Tum, R. 1984. *I, Rigoberta Menchú: An Indian woman in Guatemala.* Verso; Lovell, W. G. 2010. *A beauty that hurts: Life and death in Guatemala.* University of Texas Press; Sanford, V., and Barbour, A. 2003. *Buried secrets: Truth and human rights in Guatemala.* Palgrave Macmillan; Green, L. 1999. *Fear as a way of life: Mayan widows in rural Guatemala.* Columbia University Press; Carmack, R. M. 1988. *Harvest of violence: The Maya Indians and the Guatemalan crisis.* University of Oklahoma Press.

45. Oficina de Derechos Humanos del Arzobispado de Guatemala. 1998. *Guatemala: nunca más. Impactos de la violencia.* ODHAG.

46. Comisión para el Esclarecimiento Histórico (Guatemala). 2012. *Memory of silence: The Guatemalan truth commission report.*

47. World Bank. 2018. *Intentional homicides (per 100,000 people)—Guatemala,* accessed March 3, 2022, https://data.worldbank.org/indicator/VC.IHR.PSRC.P5?locations=GT.

48. Clouser, R. 2019. Security, development, and fear in Guatemala: Enduring ties and lasting consequences. *Geographical Review,* 109(3): 382–398.

49. Richani, N. 2010. State capacity in postconflict settings: Explaining criminal violence in El Salvador and Guatemala. *Civil Wars,* 12(4): 431–455; Tellman, B., McSweeney, K., Manak, L., Devine, J. A., Sesnie, S., Nielsen, E., and Dávila, A. 2021. Narcotrafficking and land control in Guatemala and Honduras. *Journal of Illicit Economies and Development,* 3(1).

50. Oficina de Derechos Humanos del Arzobispado de Guatemala. 1998. *Guatemala: nunca más. Impactos de la violencia.* ODHAG.

51. Goldman, F. 2010. The Art of Political Murder: Who Killed Bishop Gerardi?. Atlantic Books Ltd.

52. Nash, J. C. 2006. *Practicing ethnography in a globalizing world: An anthropological odyssey.* Rowman Altamira.

53. Transparency International. 2021. Corruption Perceptions Index for 2020: Results at a glance. *Transparency.org,* accessed March 10, 2022, https://www.transparency.org/en/cpi/2020/index/gtm.

54. Kleinman, A. 1997. "Everything that really matters": Social suffering, subjectivity, and the remaking of human experience in a disordering world. *Harvard Theological Review,* 90(3): 315–336.

55. Kleinman, A., Das, V., Lock, M., and Lock, M. M. 1997. *Social suffering.* University of California Press; Das, V., Kleinman, A., Lock, M. M., Ramphele, M., and Reynolds, P. 2001. *Remaking a world: Violence, social suffering, and recovery.* University of California Press.

56. Wilkinson, I. 2004. The problem of "social suffering": The challenge to social science. *Health Sociology Review,* 13: 113–121; Wilkinson, I. 2006. Health, risk and

"social suffering." *Health, Risk & Society*, 8(1): 1–8; Biehl, J. 2016. Theorizing global health. *Medicine Anthropology Theory*, 3; Carmack, R. M. 1988. *Harvest of violence: The Maya Indians and the Guatemalan crisis*. University of Oklahoma Press.

57. Hale, C. R. 2002. Does multiculturalism menace? Governance, cultural rights and the politics of identity in Guatemala. *Journal of Latin American Studies*, 34: 485–524.

58. Nelson, D. M. 1999. *A finger in the wound: Body politics in quincentennial Guatemala*. University of California Press.

59. Nelson, D. M. 1999. *A finger in the wound: Body politics in quincentennial Guatemala*. University of California Press; Reeves, R. 2006. *Ladinos with Ladinos, Indians with Indians: Land, labor, and regional ethnic conflict in the making of Guatemala*. Stanford University Press.

60. Arzú, M. E. C. 2002. *La metamorfosis del racismo en Guatemala*. Cholsamaj Fundacion.

61. Addiss, D. G., and Amon, J. J. 2019. Apology and unintended harm in global health. *Health and Human Rights*, 21(1): 19.

62. Hall-Clifford, R., Addiss, D. G., Cook-Deegan, R. and Lavery, J. V. 2019. Global health fieldwork ethics: Mapping the challenges. *Health and Human Rights*, 21(1): 1.

63. Spradley, J. P. 2016. *Participant observation*. Waveland Press.

64. Faubion, J. D. and Marcus, G. E. 2009. *Fieldwork is not what it used to be: Learning anthropology's method in a time of transition*. Cornell University Press.; McLean, A., and Leibing, A. (Eds.). 2008. *The shadow side of fieldwork: Exploring the blurred borders between ethnography and life*. John Wiley & Sons; Hall-Clifford, R., and Cook-Deegan, R. 2019. Ethically managing risks in global health fieldwork: Human rights ideals confront real world challenges. *Health and Human Rights*, 21(1): 7.

65. Rappaport, J. 2008. Beyond participant observation: Collaborative ethnography as theoretical innovation. *Collaborative Anthropologies*, 1(1): 1–31.

66. Hall-Clifford, R. 2022. Can co-design promote equity in global health? Speaking of medicine. *PLoS Global Public Health*. https://speakingofmedicine.plos.org/2022/11/15/can-co-design-promote-equity-in-global-health/.

67. Hall-Clifford, R., and Amerson, R. 2017. From guidelines to local realities: Evaluation of oral rehydration therapy and zinc supplementation in Guatemala. *Revista Panamericana de Salud Publica*, 41: e8; Amerson, R., Hall-Clifford, R., Thompson, B., and Comninellas, N. 2015. Implementation of a training program for low-literacy promotoras in oral rehydration therapy. *Public Health Nursing*, 32(2): 177–185.

68. Martinez, B., Hall-Clifford, R., Coyote, E., Stroux, L., Valderrama, C. E., Aaron, C., Francis, A., Hendren, C., Rohloff, P., and Clifford, G. D. 2017. Agile development of a smartphone app for perinatal monitoring in a resource-constrained setting.

Journal of Health Informatics in Developing Countries, 11(1); Martinez, B., Ixen, E. C., Hall-Clifford, R., Juarez, M., Miller, A. C., Francis, A., Valderrama, C. E., Stroux, L., Clifford, G. D., and Rohloff, P. 2018. mHealth intervention to improve the continuum of maternal and perinatal care in rural Guatemala: A pragmatic, randomized controlled feasibility trial. *Reproductive Health*, 15: 1–12.

69. Walford, G. 2018. The impossibility of anonymity in ethnographic research. *Qualitative Research*, 18(5): 516–525.

70. Lassiter, L. 2005. Collaborative ethnography and public anthropology. *Current Anthropology*, 46(1): 83–106; Rappaport, J. 2008. Beyond participant observation: Collaborative ethnography as theoretical innovation. *Collaborative Anthropologies*, 1(1): 1–31.

71. Graham, A. 2014. One hundred years of suffering? "Humanitarian crisis photography" and self-representation in the Democratic Republic of the Congo. *Social Dynamics*, 40(1), 140–163; Graham, A. P., Lavery, J. V., and Cook-Deegan, R. 2019. Ethics of global health photography: A focus on being more human. *Health and Human Rights*, 21(1): 49.

72. Hale, C. R. 2002. Does multiculturalism menace? Governance, cultural rights and the politics of identity in Guatemala. *Journal of Latin American Studies*, 34: 485–524; Hale, C. 2006. *Más que un indio: Racial Ambivalence and the Paradox of Neoliberal Multiculturalism in Guatemala*. School of American Research Press.

73. Steltzer, U. 1983. *Health in the Guatemalan highlands*. University of Washington Press.

74. Stoll, D. 1993. *Between two armies in the Ixil towns of Guatemala*. Columbia University Press; Heggenhougen, H. K. 1984. Will primary health care efforts be allowed to succeed? *Social Science & Medicine*, 19: 217–224.

75. Hale, C. R. 2002. Does multiculturalism menace? Governance, cultural rights and the politics of identity in Guatemala. *Journal of Latin American Studies*, 34: 485–524.

76. Maupin, J. N. 2009. "Fruit of the accords": Healthcare reform and civil participation in highland Guatemala. *Social Science & Medicine*, 68(8): 1456–1463.

77. Pan American Health Organization (PAHO). 2017. *Health in the Americas: Guatemala country report*, accessed March 10, 2022, https://www.paho.org/salud-en-las-americas-2017.

Chapter 1

1. Steltzer, U. 1983. *Health in the Guatemalan highlands*. University of Washington Press; Hall-Clifford, R., and Amerson, R. 2017. From guidelines to local realities: Evaluation of oral rehydration therapy and zinc supplementation in Guatemala. *Revista Panamericana de Salud Publica*, 41: e8.

2. Hall-Clifford, R. A. 2009. *Oral rehydration therapy in highland Guatemala: Long-term impacts of public health intervention on the self.* Boston University.

3. Polgar, S. 1963. Health action in cross-cultural perspective. In *Handbook of medical sociology*, Freeman, H.E., Levine, S., and Reeder, L.G., eds. Prentice-Hall. 397–419.

4. World Health Organization. 2017. *Diarrhoeal disease*, accessed February 19, 2022, https://www.who.int/news-room/fact-sheets/detail/diarrhoeal-disease.

5. Diarrhea can also have noninfectious causes, such as certain medications, diet, and chronic health conditions.

6. Bentley, M. E., Pelto, G. H., Straus, W. L., Schumann, D. A., Adegbola, C., de la Pena, E., Oni, G. A., Brown, K. H., and Huffman, S. L. 1988. Rapid ethnographic assessment: Applications in a diarrhea management program. Special issue, *Social Science & Medicine*, 27(1): 107–116. https://doi.org/10.1016/0277-9536(88)90168-2.

7. Cordon, A., Asturias, G., De Vries, T., and Rohloff, P. 2019. Advancing child nutrition science in the scaling up nutrition era: A systematic scoping review of stunting research in Guatemala. *BMJ Paediatrics Open*, 3(1); Chary, A., Messmer, S., Sorenson, E., Henretty, N., Dasgupta, S., and Rohloff, P. 2013. The normalization of childhood disease: An ethnographic study of child malnutrition in rural Guatemala. *Human Organization*, 72(2): 87–97.

8. Maung, K. U., and Greenough, W. B. 1991. Treatment of the dehydrated child. *Pediatric annals*, 20(1).

9. Cash, R. A. 1983. Oral rehydration in the treatment of diarrhea: Issues in the implementation of diarrhea treatment programs. 203–221 In L. C. Chen and N. S. Scrimshaw (Eds.), *Diarrhea and malnutrition: Interactions, mechanisms, and interventions.* Springer London: Plenum Press.

10. Maung, K. U., and Greenough, W. B. 1991. Treatment of the dehydrated child. *Pediatric annals*, 20(1); Ruxin, J. N. 1994. Magic bullet: the history of oral rehydration therapy. *Medical History*, 38(4): 363–397.

11. The updated formula reduced osmolarity to improve absorption through the endothelial lining of the small intestine.

12. Wolfheim, C., Fontaine, O., and Merson, M. 2019. Evolution of the World Health Organization's programmatic actions to control diarrheal diseases. *Journal of Global Health*, 9: 020802. https://doi.org/10.7189/jogh.09.020802.

13. Perry, H. B., Zulliger, R., and Rogers, M. M. 2014. Community health workers in low-, middle-, and high-income countries: An overview of their history, recent evolution, and current effectiveness. *Annual Review of Public Health*, 35: 399–421; Perry, H. B., and Zulliger, R. 2012. How effective are community health workers? Technical report. Johns Hopkins Bloomberg School of Public Health; Liu, A., Sullivan, S., Khan,

M., Sachs, S., and Singh, P. 2011. Community health workers in global health: Scale and scalability. *Mount Sinai Journal of Medicine: A Journal of Translational and Personalized Medicine*, 78: 419–435.

14. Maung, K. U., and Greenough, W. B. 1991. Treatment of the dehydrated child. *Pediatric annals*, 20(1); Snyder, J. D., Molla, A. M., and Cash, R. A. 1990. Home-based therapy for diarrhea. *Journal of Pediatric Gastroenterology and Nutrition*, 11: 438–447.

15. Cash, R. A. 1983. Oral rehydration in the treatment of diarrhea: Issues in the implementation of diarrhea treatment programs. In *Diarrhea and malnutrition*. Springer, 203–221; Nalin, D. R., and Cash, R. A. 2018. 50 years of oral rehydration therapy: The solution is still simple. *The Lancet*, 392: 536–538.

16. Cash, R. A. 1983. Oral rehydration in the treatment of diarrhea: Issues in the implementation of diarrhea treatment programs. In *Diarrhea and malnutrition*, 203–221. Springer; Nalin, D. R., and Cash, R. A. 2018. 50 years of oral rehydration therapy: The solution is still simple. *The Lancet*, 392: 536–538.

17. World Health Organization. 1993. *The management and prevention of diarrhoea: Practical guidelines*. WHO; Ruxin, J. N. 1994. Magic bullet: The history of oral rehydration therapy. *Medical History*, 38(4): 363–397.

18. Suh, J.-S., Hahn, W.-H., and Cho, B.-S. 2010. Recent advances of oral rehydration therapy (ORT). *Electrolytes & Blood Pressure*, 8: 82–86; World Health Organization. 2006. *Oral rehydration salts: Production of the new solution*. WHO. https://www.who.int/publications/i/item/WHO-FCH-CAH-06.1; Maung, K. U., and Greenough, W. B. 1991. Treatment of the dehydrated child. *Pediatric annals*, 20(1).

19. Gracey, M. 1997. Diarrheal disease in perspective. In M. Gracey and J. A. Walker-Smith (Eds.), *Diarrheal disease*. Nestle Nutrition Services.

20. Gracey, M. 1997. Diarrheal disease in perspective. In M. Gracey and J. A. Walker-Smith (Eds.), *Diarrheal disease*. Nestle Nutrition Services.

21. World Health Organization. 2017. *Diarrhoeal disease*, accessed February 19, 2022, https://www.who.int/news-room/fact-sheets/detail/diarrhoeal-disease.

22. Das, J. K., Salam, R. A., and Bhutta, Z. A. 2014. Global burden of childhood diarrhea and interventions. *Current Opinion in Infectious Diseases*, 27: 451–458; Boschi-Pinto, C., Lanata, C. F., and Black, R. E. 2009. The global burden of childhood diarrhea. In *Maternal and child health*, 225–243. Springer.

23. Cash, R. A. 2021. Using oral rehydration therapy (ORT) in the community. *Tropical Medicine and Infectious Disease*, 6(2): 92; Ezezika, O., Ragunathan, A., El-Bakri, Y., and Barrett, K. 2021. Barriers and facilitators to implementation of oral rehydration therapy in low-and middle-income countries: A systematic review. *PLoS One*, 16(4): e0249638.

24. Greenough III, W. B. 1991. Cereal-based oral rehydration therapy. I. Clinical studies. *Journal of Pediatrics*, 118: S72–S79; Molla, A. M., Khapam, A., Molla, A., Eeckels, R., and Greenough III, W. B. 1985. Comparison of efficacy and digestibility of plantain-salt and rice-salt as home fluid with standard glucose ORS in the management of rehydration in acute diarrhoea in children, Research report accessed at: http://dspace.icddrb .org/jspui/bitstream/123456789/755/1/ICDDRBProtocol-1985-019.pdf, Accessed on 15 July 2023; Farthing, M., Salam, M. A., Lindberg, G., Dite, P., Khalif, I., Salazar-Lindo, E., Ramakrishna, B. S., Goh, K.-L., Thomson, A., Khan, A. G., Krabshuis, J., LeMair, A., and WGO. 2013. Acute diarrhea in adults and children: A global perspective. *Journal of Clinical Gastroenterology*, 47: 12–20. https://doi.org/10.1097/MCG.0b013e31826df662; Nations, M. K., and Rebhun, L.-A. 1988. Mystification of a simple solution: Oral rehydration therapy in Northeast Brazil. *Social Science & Medicine*, 27: 25–38.

25. World Health Organization. 2005. *The treatment of diarrhoea*. WHO.

26. Nations, M. K., and Rebhun, L.-A. 1988. Mystification of a simple solution: Oral rehydration therapy in Northeast Brazil. *Social Science & Medicine*, 27: 25–38.

27. World Health Organization. 1993. *The management and prevention of diarrhoea: Practical guidelines*. WHO; Snyder, J. D., Molla, A. M., and Cash, R. A. 1990. Home-based therapy for diarrhea. *Journal of Pediatric Gastroenterology and Nutrition*, 11: 438–447.

28. Greenbough, W. B., and Khin-Maung-U. 1991. Rehydration therapy. In *Diarrheal diseases*. London: Elsevier.

29. Wagner, Z., Asiimwe, J. B., Dow, W. H., and Levine, D. I. 2019. The role of price and convenience in use of oral rehydration salts to treat child diarrhea: A cluster randomized trial in Uganda. *PLoS Medicine*, 16: e1002734. https://doi.org/10.1371 /journal.pmed.1002734; Hall-Clifford, R., and Amerson, R. 2017. From guidelines to local realities: Evaluation of oral rehydration therapy and zinc supplementation in Guatemala. *Revista Panamericana de Salud Publica*, 41: e8.

30. World Health Organization. 1993. *The management and prevention of diarrhoea: Practical guidelines*. WHO; Cash, R. A. 1983. Oral rehydration in the treatment of diarrhea: Issues in the implementation of diarrhea treatment programs. In *Diarrhea and malnutrition*. Springer, 203–221.

31. United Nations Millennium Development Goals. n.d. *Goal 7: Ensure environmental sustainability*, accessed March 10, 2022, https://www.un.org/millenniumgoals /environ.shtml.

32. World Bank. 2018. Guatemala's water supply, sanitation, and hygiene poverty diagnostic. Technical report. World Bank Group.

33. World Bank. 2018. Guatemala's water supply, sanitation, and hygiene poverty diagnostic. Technical report. World Bank Group.

34. Trudeau, J., Aksan, A.-M., and Vásquez, W. F. 2018. Water system unreliability and diarrhea incidence among children in Guatemala. *International Journal of Public Health*, 63: 241–250. https://doi.org/10.1007/s00038-017-1054-6.

35. Darvesh, N., Das, J. K., Vaivada, T., Gaffey, M. F., Rasanathan, K., Bhutta, Z. A., and Social Determinants of Health Study Team. 2017. Water, sanitation and hygiene interventions for acute childhood diarrhea: A systematic review to provide estimates for the Lives Saved Tool. *BMC Public Health*, 17: 776. https://doi.org/10.1186/s12889 -017-4746-1; Vásquez, W. F. 2011. Municipal water services in Guatemala: Exploring official perceptions. *Water Policy*, 13: 362–374.

36. Banerjee, O., Cicowiez, M., Horridge, M., and Vargas, R. 2019. Evaluating synergies and trade-offs in achieving the SDGs of zero hunger and clean water and sanitation: An application of the IEEM Platform to Guatemala. *Ecological Economics*, 161: 280–291.

37. Heuveline, P., and Goldman, N. 2000. A description of child illness and treatment behavior in Guatemala. *Social Science & Medicine*, 50: 345–364; Kumar, V., Kumar, R., and Raina, N. 1989. Impact of oral rehydration therapy on maternal beliefs and practices related to acute diarrhea. *Indian Journal of Pediatrics*, 56: 219–225. https://doi.org/10.1007/BF02726612.

38. Fischer Walker, C. L., Fontaine, O., Young, M. W., and Black, R. E. 2009. Zinc and low osmolarity oral rehydration salts for diarrhoea: A renewed call to action. *Bulletin of the World Health Organization*, 87: 780–786. https://doi.org/10.2471/blt.08 .058990.

39. Santosham, M., Chandran, A., Fitzwater, S., Fischer-Walker, C., Baqui, A. H., and Black, R. 2010. Progress and barriers for the control of diarrhoeal disease. *The Lancet*, 376: 63–67. https://doi.org/10.1016/S0140-6736(10)60356-X; Lamberti, L. M., Walker, C. L. F., Chan, K. Y., Jian, W.-Y., and Black, R. E. 2013. Oral zinc supplementation for the treatment of acute diarrhea in children: A systematic review and meta-analysis. *Nutrients*, 5: 4715–4740. https://doi.org/10.3390/nu5114715; World Health Organization. 2005. *The treatment of diarrhoea*. WHO.

40. Government of the Republic of Guatemala. 2017. *Consejo Nacional de Seguridad Alimentaria y Nutricional*. Technical report. Gobierno De La Republica de Guatemala.

41. Roche, M., García Meza, R., and Vossenaar, M. 2015. An intervention to co-package zinc and oral rehydration salts (ORS) improves health provider prescription and maternal adherence to WHO-recommended diarrhea treatment in Western Guatemala. *FASEB Journal*, 29: 902.23.

42. García Meza, R., Roche, M., Vossenaar, M., and Solomons, N. 2015. Maternal perceptions and experiences with an intervention to increase adherence to WHO-recommended zinc (Zn)+oral rehydration salts (ORS) for diarrhea treatment in Western Guatemala. *FASEB Journal*, 29: 584.19.

43. Hall-Clifford, R., and Amerson, R. 2017. From guidelines to local realities: Evaluation of oral rehydration therapy and zinc supplementation in Guatemala. *Revista Panamericana de Salud Publica*, 41: e8.

44. World Health Organization. 2005. *The treatment of diarrhoea*. WHO.

45. Instituto Guatemalteco de Seguridad Social. 2014. *Plan Operativo Anual Institucional y Presupuesto 2014*. Instituto Guatemalteco de Seguridad Social.

46. Kragel, E. A., Merz, A., Flood, D. M. N., and Haven, K. E. 2020. Risk factors for stunting in children under the age of 5 in rural Guatemalan highlands. *Annals of Global Health*, 86: 8. https://doi.org/10.5334/aogh.2433.

47. Walson, J. L., and Berkley, J. A. 2018. The impact of malnutrition on childhood infections. *Current Opinion in Infectious Diseases*, 31: 231–236. https://doi.org/10.1097/QCO.0000000000000448; Bogin, B., Silva, M. I. V., and Rios, L. 2007. Life history trade-offs in human growth: Adaptation or pathology? *American Journal of Human Biology*, 19: 631–642. https://doi.org/10.1002/ajhb.20666; Goudet, S., Griffiths, P., Bogin, B., and Madise, N. 2017. Interventions to tackle malnutrition and its risk factors in children living in slums: A scoping review. *Annals of Human Biology*, 44: 1–10. https://doi.org/10.1080/03014460.2016.1205660.

48. Bogin, B. 2022. Fear, violence, inequality, and stunting in Guatemala. *American Journal of Human Biology*, 34: e23627. https://doi.org/10.1002/ajhb.23627.

49. Chary, A., Messmer, S., Sorenson, E., Henretty, N., Dasgupta, S., and Rohloff, P. 2013. The normalization of childhood disease: An ethnographic study of child malnutrition in rural Guatemala. *Human Organization*, 72(2): 87–97; Rohloff, P. 2021. On the frontlines of chronic paediatric undernutrition in Guatemala. *eBioMedicine*, 64: 103223. https://doi.org/10.1016/j.ebiom.2021.103223.

50. Hall-Clifford, R. A. 2009. *Oral rehydration therapy in highland Guatemala: Long-term impacts of public health intervention on the self* (Doctoral dissertation), Boston University; Hall-Clifford, R., and Amerson, R. 2017. From guidelines to local realities: Evaluation of oral rehydration therapy and zinc supplementation in Guatemala. *Revista Panamericana de Salud Publica*, 41: e8.

51. Pebley, A., Hurtado, E., and Goldman, N. 1999. Beliefs about children's illness. *Journal of Biosocial Science*, 31: 195–219.

52. Kleinman, A. 1980. *Patients and healers in the context of culture*. University of California Press.

53. Nigenda, G., Mora-Flores, G., Aldama-López, S., and Orozco-Núñez, E. 2001. Practice of traditional medicine in Latin America and the Caribbean: The dilemma between regulation and tolerance. *Salud Pública de México*, 43: 41–51.

54. Chary, A., and Rohloff, P. (Eds.). 2015. *Privatization and the new medical pluralism: Shifting healthcare landscapes in Maya Guatemala*. Lexington Books.

55. Foster, G. M. 1994. *Hippocrates' Latin American legacy: Humoral medicine in the New World*. Taylor & Francis.

56. Foster, G. M. 1994. *Hippocrates' Latin American legacy: Humoral medicine in the New World*. Taylor & Francis.

57. Foster, G. M. 1994. *Hippocrates' Latin American legacy: Humoral medicine in the New World*. Taylor & Francis.

58. I use George Foster's method of distinguishing metaphoric Hot and Cold (with capital letters) from thermal temperatures, all four of which are distinguished in the humoral systems discussed.

59. Foster, G. M. 1994. *Hippocrates' Latin American legacy: Humoral medicine in the New World*. Taylor & Francis.

60. Burleigh, E., Dardano, C., and Cruz, J. R. 1990. Colors, humors, and evil eye: Indigenous classification and treatment of childhood diarrhea in highland Guatemala. *Medical Anthropology*, 12: 419–441.

61. Pebley, A., Hurtado, E., and Goldman, N. 1999. Beliefs about children's illness. *Journal of Biosocial Science*, 31: 195–219.

62. Pebley, A., Hurtado, E. and Goldman, N. 1999. Beliefs about children's illness. *Journal of Biosocial Science*, 31: 195–219.

63. Pebley, A., Hurtado, E. and Goldman, N. 1999. Beliefs about children's illness. *Journal of Biosocial Science*, 31: 195–219.

64. Pebley, A., Hurtado, E., and Goldman, N. 1999. Beliefs about children's illness. *Journal of Biosocial Science*, 31: 195–219.

65. Douglas, M. 1973. *Natural symbols: Explorations in cosmology*. Barrie and Jenkins see also Douglas, M. 1966. *Purity and danger: An analysis of the concepts of pollution and taboo*. Routledge, 98–99.

66. Tedlock, B. 1987. An interpretive solution to the problem of humoral medicine in Latin America. *Social Science & Medicine* 24: 1069–1083; Foster, G. M. 1994. *Hippocrates' Latin American legacy: Humoral medicine in the New World*. Taylor & Francis.

67. Nigenda, G., Mora-Flores, G., Aldama-López, S., and Orozco-Núñez, E. 2001. Practice of traditional medicine in Latin America and the Caribbean: The dilemma between regulation and tolerance. *Salud Pública de México*, 43: 41–51; Huff, R. M. 2020. Traditional healing practices and healers. In *The Wiley Encyclopedia of Health Psychology*, 199–204. Wiley; Montenegro, R. A., and Stephens, C. 2006. Indigenous health in Latin America and the Caribbean. *The Lancet*, 367: 1859–1869. https://doi.org/10.1016/S0140-6736(06)68808-9.

68. Foster, G. M. 1994. *Hippocrates' Latin American legacy: Humoral medicine in the New World*. Taylor & Francis.

69. Kendall, C., Foote, D., and Martorell, R. 1984. Ethnomedicine and oral rehydration therapy: A case study of ethnomedical investigation and program planning. *Social Science & Medicine*, 19: 253–260.

70. Kendall, C., Foote, D., and Martorell, R. 1984. Ethnomedicine and oral rehydration therapy: A case study of ethnomedical investigation and program planning. *Social Science & Medicine*, 19: 253–260.

71. Hall-Clifford, R. A. 2009. *Oral rehydration therapy in highland Guatemala: Long-term impacts of public health intervention on the self* (Doctoral dissertation), Boston University; Hall-Clifford, R., and Amerson, R. 2017. From guidelines to local realities: Evaluation of oral rehydration therapy and zinc supplementation in Guatemala. *Revista Panamericana de Salud Publica*, 41: e8.

72. Burleigh, E., Dardano, C., and Cruz, J. R. 1990. Colors, humors, and evil eye: Indigenous classification and treatment of childhood diarrhea in highland Guatemala. *Medical Anthropology*, 12: 419–441.

73. Burleigh, E., Dardano, C., and Cruz, J. R. 1990. Colors, humors, and evil eye: Indigenous classification and treatment of childhood diarrhea in highland Guatemala. *Medical Anthropology*, 12: 419–441.

74. Burleigh, E., Dardano, C., and Cruz, J. R. 1990. Colors, humors, and evil eye: Indigenous classification and treatment of childhood diarrhea in highland Guatemala. *Medical Anthropology*, 12: 419–441; Kendall, C., Foote, D., and Martorell, R. 1984. Ethnomedicine and oral rehydration therapy: A case study of ethnomedical investigation and program planning. *Social Science & Medicine*, 19: 253–260.

75. Hoyler, E., Martinez, R., Mehta, K., Nisonoff, H., and Boyd, D. 2018. Beyond medical pluralism: Characterising health-care delivery of biomedicine and traditional medicine in rural Guatemala. *Global Public Health*, 13(4): 503–517.

76. Werner, D., Sanders, D., and Weston, J. 1997. *Questioning the solution: The politics of primary health care and child survival, with an in-depth critique of oral rehydration therapy*. HealthWrights.

77. Edejer, T. T.-T., Aikins, M., Black, R., Wolfson, L., Hutubessy, R., and Evans, D. B. 2005. Cost effectiveness analysis of strategies for child health in developing countries. *BMJ*, 331: 1177. https://doi.org/10.1136/bmj.38652.550278.7C.

78. Local Burden of Disease Diarrhoea Collaborators. 2020. Mapping geographical inequalities in oral rehydration therapy coverage in low-income and middle-income countries, 2000–17. *The Lancet Global Health*, 8: e1038–e1060. https://doi.org/10.1016/S2214-109X(20)30230-8.

79. Local Burden of Disease Diarrhoea Collaborators. 2020. Mapping geographical inequalities in oral rehydration therapy coverage in low-income and middle-income countries, 2000–17. *The Lancet Global Health*, 8: e1038–e1060. https://doi.org/10.1016/S2214-109X(20)30230-8.

80. World Bank. 2020. *Poverty and equity brief: Latin America and the Caribbean—Guatemala*. World Bank Group.

81. Werner, D., Sanders, D., and Weston, J. 1997. *Questioning the solution: The politics of primary health care and child survival, with an in-depth critique of oral rehydration therapy*. HealthWrights.

82. Hall-Clifford, R. A. 2009. *Oral rehydration therapy in highland Guatemala: Long-term impacts of public health intervention on the self* (Doctoral dissertation), Boston University.

83. Douglas, M. 1973. *Natural symbols: Explorations in cosmology*. Routledge.

84. Wade, L. 2010. Colonialism, soap, and the cleansing metaphor—sociological images. *The Society Pages*, accessed March 10, 2022, https://thesocietypages.org/socimages/2010/08/10/colonialism-soap-and-the-cleansing-metaphor/.

Chapter 2

1. Hall-Clifford, R., and Amerson, R. 2017. From guidelines to local realities: Evaluation of oral rehydration therapy and zinc supplementation in Guatemala. *Revista Panamericana de Salud Publica*, 41: e8.

2. Menjívar, C. 2011. *Enduring violence: Ladina women's lives in Guatemala*. University of California Press.

3. Nelson, D. M. 1999. *A finger in the wound: Body politics in quincentennial Guatemala*. University of California Press.

4. Nelson, D. M. 1999. *A finger in the wound: Body politics in quincentennial Guatemala*. University of California Press; Berger, S. 2006, *Guatemaltecas: The women's movement, 1986–2003*. University of Texas Press.

5. Bennett, J. N. 2022. *Good Maya women: Migration and revitalization of clothing and language in highland Guatemala*. University of Alabama Press.

6. Nelson, D. M. 1999. *A finger in the wound: Body politics in quincentennial Guatemala*. University of California Press.

7. Menjívar, C. 2011. *Enduring violence: Ladina women's lives in Guatemala*. University of California Press.

8. Nelson, D. M. 1999. *A finger in the wound: Body politics in quincentennial Guatemala*. University of California Press.

9. Stern, M. 2005. *Naming security—constructing identity: "Mayan women" in Guatemala on the eve of "peace."* Manchester University Press; Torres, M. G. 2015. Gender-based violence and the state in Guatemala's genocide and beyond. In J. R. Wies and H. J. Haldane (Eds.), *Applying anthropology to gender-based violence: Global responses, local practices*. Lexington Books.

10. Infosegura. 2021. *Violence against women, Guatemala 2020*, accessed June 1, 2022, https://infosegura.org/en/2021/06/18/violence-against-women-guatemala-2020/.

11. Infosegura. 2021. *Violence against women, Guatemala 2020*, accessed June 1, 2022, https://infosegura.org/en/2021/06/18/violence-against-women-guatemala-2020/.

12. Amnesty International Guatemala. 2011. *Guatemala must act to stop the killing of women*, accessed May 30, 2022, https://www.amnesty.org/en/latest/news/2011/03 /guatemala-must-act-stop-killing-women/.

13. Amnesty International Guatemala. 2005. *No protection, no justice: Killings of women in Guatemala*, accessed June 1, 2022, https://www.amnesty.org/en/wp-content/uploads /2021/08/amr340192006en.pdf.

14. Blenford, A. 2005. Guatemala's epidemic of killing. *BBC News*, accessed June 9, 2022, http://news.bbc.co.uk/1/hi/world/americas/4074880.stm.

15. Nelson, D. M. 1999. *A finger in the wound: Body politics in quincentennial Guatemala*. University of California Press.

16. DiGeorgio-Lutz, J., and Mandujano, M. C. G. 2020. Genocide memorialization and gendered remembrance in Guatemala and Cambodia. In *Remembrance and forgiveness*, 85–97. Routledge.

17. Torres, M. G. 2015. Gender-based violence and the state in Guatemala's genocide and beyond. In J. R. Wies and H. J. Haldane (Eds.), *Applying anthropology to gender-based violence: Global responses, local practices*. Lexington Books.

18. Blenford, A. 2005. Guatemala's epidemic of killing. *BBC News*, accessed June 9, 2022, http://news.bbc.co.uk/1/hi/world/americas/4074880.stm.

19. Amnesty International Guatemala. 2005. *No protection, no justice: Killings of women in Guatemala*, accessed June 1, 2022, https://www.amnesty.org/en/wp-content /uploads/2021/08/amr340192006en.pdf.

20. UN Women. 2014. *Guatemala*, accessed May 30, 2022, https://lac.unwomen.org /en/donde-estamos/guatemala.

21. Berger, S. 2006. *Guatemaltecas: The women's movement, 1986–2003*. University of Texas Press; Menjívar, C. 2011. *Enduring violence: Ladina women's lives in Guatemala*. University of California Press.

22. Sanford, V. 2007. Memories of a friend in the field: Justice for Pepe, justice for Guatemala. *Anthropology News*, 48(7): 26.

23. UN Women. 2014. *Guatemala*, accessed May 30, 2022, https://lac.unwomen.org /en/donde-estamos/guatemala.

24. UN Women. 2014. *Guatemala*, accessed May 30, 2022, https://lac.unwomen.org /en/donde-estamos/guatemala.

25. Fischer, E. F., and Benson, P. 2006. *Broccoli and desire: Global connections and Maya struggles in postwar Guatemala*. Stanford University Press.

26. World Bank. 2021. *Literacy rate, youth female (% of females ages 15–24)—Guatemala*, accessed May 30, 2022, https://data.worldbank.org/indicator/SE.ADT.1524.LT.FE.ZS ?locations=GT; UN Women. 2014. *Guatemala*, accessed May 30, 2022, https://lac .unwomen.org/en/donde-estamos/guatemala.

27. Little, W. E. 2004. *Mayas in the marketplace: Tourism, globalization, and cultural identity*. University of Texas Press.

28. *Incaparina* is the most popular brand of atol beverage, created and marketed by INCAP (Institute of Nutrition for Central America and Panama).

29. Burleigh, E., Dardano, C., and Cruz, J. R. 1990. Colors, humors and evil eye: Indigenous classification and treatment of childhood diarrhea in highland Guatemala, *Medical Anthropology*, 12(1): 419–441. https://doi.org/10.1080/01459740.1990 .9966035; Heuveline, P., and Goldman, N. 2000. A description of child illness and treatment behavior in Guatemala. *Social Science & Medicine*, 50: 345–364.

30. Burleigh, E., Dardano, C., and Cruz, J. R. 1990. Colors, humors and evil eye: Indigenous classification and treatment of childhood diarrhea in highland Guatemala, *Medical Anthropology*, 12(1): 419–441. https://doi.org/10.1080/01459740.1990 .9966035.

31. Chary, A., Messmer, S., Sorenson, E., Henretty, N., Dasgupta, S., and Rohloff, P. 2013. The normalization of childhood disease: An ethnographic study of child malnutrition in rural Guatemala. *Human Organization*, 72(2): 87–97.

32. In keeping with the mentality to waste nothing, after the egg had served its purpose as a diarrheal treatment, it was cooked and eaten at dinner.

33. Maupin, J. N. 2009. "Fruit of the accords": Healthcare reform and civil participation in highland Guatemala. *Social Science & Medicine*, 68(8): 1456–1463; Berry, N. S. 2010. *Unsafe motherhood: Mayan maternal mortality and subjectivity in post-war Guatemala*. Berghahn Books; Cosminsky, S. 2016. *Midwives and mothers: The medicalization of childbirth on a Guatemalan plantation*. University of Texas Press.

34. Hall-Clifford, R. A. 2009. *Oral rehydration therapy in highland Guatemala: Long-term impacts of public health intervention on the self* (Doctoral dissertation), Boston University.

35. Hall-Clifford, R. A. 2009. *Oral rehydration therapy in highland Guatemala: Long-term impacts of public health intervention on the self* (Doctoral dissertation), Boston University.

36. Cash, R. A. 1983. Oral rehydration in the treatment of diarrhea: Issues in the implementation of diarrhea treatment programs. In L. C. Chen and N. S. Scrimshaw

(Eds.), *Diarrhea and malnutrition: Interactions, mechanisms, and interventions*. Plenum Press.

37. Cash, R. A. 1983. Oral rehydration in the treatment of diarrhea: Issues in the implementation of diarrhea treatment programs. In L. C. Chen and N. S. Scrimshaw (Eds.), *Diarrhea and malnutrition: Interactions, mechanisms, and interventions*. Plenum Press; Gracey, M. 1985. The WHO diarrhoeal diseases control programme. In M. Gracey (Ed.), *Diarrhoeal disease and malnutrition: A clinical update*. Churchill Livingstone; Gracey, M. 1997. Diarrheal disease in perspective. In M. Gracey and J. A. Walker-Smith (Eds.), *Diarrheal disease*. Nestle Nutrition Services.

38. Morales, M. S. 2004. *Informe Final de Investigación Epidemiológica: Factores de Riesgo Asociados a Morbilidad por Diarrea en Niños de Cinco Años de San Juan Comalapa, Chimaltenango*. Universidad de San Carlos.

39. Brettell, C. B. 1998. Historical perspectives on infant and child mortality in northwestern Portugal. In *Small wars: The cultural politics of childhood*, 165–185. Scheper-Hughes, N., & Sargent, C. F. (Eds.). (1998). *Small wars: The cultural politics of childhood*. Univ of California Press.

40. Wehr, H., Chary, A., Webb, M. F., and Rohloff, P. 2014. Implications of gender and household roles in Indigenous Maya communities in Guatemala for child nutrition interventions. *International Journal of Indigenous Health*, 10(1): 100–113.

41. Engle, P. L., and Nieves, I. 1993. Intra-household food distribution among Guatemalan families in a supplementary feeding program: behavior patterns. *Social Science & Medicine*, 36(12): 1605–1612.

42. Tumilowicz, A., Habicht, J. P., Pelto, G., and Pelletier, D. L. 2015. Gender perceptions predict sex differences in growth patterns of Indigenous Guatemalan infants and young children. *American Journal of Clinical Nutrition*, 102(5): 1249–1258.

43. World Bank. 2015. *Contraceptive prevalence, any modern method (% of married women ages 15–49)—Guatemala*. https://data.worldbank.org/indicator/SP.DYN.CONM .ZS?locations=GT.

44. The conversation was held primarily in Kaqchikel Maya, with some Spanish when participants switched. My research assistant Myrna, who helped facilitate during some discussions, transcribed the recording into Spanish, and I have translated to English.

45. Richardson, E., Allison, K. R., Gesink, D., and Berry, A. 2016. Barriers to accessing and using contraception in highland Guatemala: The development of a family planning self-efficacy scale. *Open Access Journal of Contraception*, 1: 77–87.

46. Heckert, C. 2018. *Fault lines of care: Gender, HIV, and global health in Bolivia*. Rutgers University Press.

47. Flood, D., Chary, A., Colom, A., and Rohloff, P. 2018. Adolescent rights and the "first 1,000 days" global nutrition movement: A view from Guatemala. *Health and Human Rights*, 20(1): 295.

48. Colom, A. 2015. Forced motherhood in Guatemala: An analysis of the thousand days initiative. In A. Chary and P. Rohloff (Eds.), *Privatization and the new medical pluralism: Shifting healthcare landscapes in Maya Guatemala*. Lexington Books.

49. Behar, R. 1997. *The vulnerable observer: Anthropology that breaks your heart*. Beacon Press.

50. Nelson, D. M. 2015. *Who counts? The mathematics of death and life after genocide*. Duke University Press.

51. Hall-Clifford, R. 2019. Where there is no hashtag: Considering gender-based violence in global health fieldwork in the time of# MeToo. *Health and Human Rights*, 21(1): 129.

52. Gifford, L., and Hall-Clifford, R. 2008. From catcalls to kidnapping: Towards an open dialogue on the fieldwork experiences of graduate women. *Anthropology News*, 49(6): 26–27; Hall-Clifford, R. 2019. Where there is no hashtag: Considering gender-based violence in global health fieldwork in the time of# MeToo. *Health and Human Rights*, 21(1): 129.

53. Hall-Clifford, R., Addiss, D., Brown, P., Castro, A., Clisbee, M., Cook-Deegan, R., Evans, D.P. et al. 2019. #MeToo meets global health: A call to action. *Health and Human Rights*, 21: 133.

54. Yates-Doerr, E. 2020. Antihero care: On fieldwork and anthropology. *Anthropology and Humanism*, 45(2): 233–244.

55. Scheper-Hughes, N. 1993. Death without weeping: The violence of everyday life in Brazil. Univ of California Press.; Biehl, J., 2013. Vita: Life in a zone of social abandonment. Univ of California Press.; Farmer, P., 2004. Pathologies of Power: Health, Human Rights, and the New War on the Poor. Univ of California Press.; Heggenhougen, H.K., 2009. Planting "Seeds of Health" in the fields of structural violence: The Ilife and death of Francisco Curruchiche. Global health in times of violence, pp.181–200.

56. Heckert, C. 2018. *Fault lines of care: Gender, HIV, and global health in Bolivia*. Rutgers University Press.

57. Global Health 50/50. 2018. *Global Health 50/50 Report*, accessed June 1, 2022, https://globalhealth5050.org/report/.

58. Carey, D. 2013. Forced and forbidden sex: Rape and sexual freedom in dictatorial Guatemala. *The Americas*, 69(3): 357–389.

59. Catino, J., Colom, A., and Ruiz, M. 2011. Equipping Mayan girls to improve their lives. *Population Council*, accessed May 30, 2022, https://knowledgecommons .popcouncil.org/departments_sbsr-pgy/803/; Flood, D., Chary, A., and Colom, A., and Rohloff, P. 2018. Adolescent rights and the "first 1,000 days" global nutrition movement: a view from Guatemala. *Health and Human Rights*, 20(1): 295–301.

60. Wehr, H., and Tum, S. E. 2013. When a girl's decision involves the community: The realities of adolescent Maya girls' lives in rural Indigenous Guatemala. *Reproductive Health Matters*, 21(41): 136–142.

61. Maes, K. C., Kohrt, B. A., and Closser, S. 2010. Culture, status and context in community health worker pay: Pitfalls and opportunities for policy research. A commentary on Glenton et al. 2010. *Social Science & Medicine*, 71(8): 1375–1378.

62. Maes, K. C., Kohrt, B. A., and Closser, S. 2010. Culture, status and context in community health worker pay: Pitfalls and opportunities for policy research. A commentary on Glenton et al. 2010. *Social Science & Medicine*, 71(8): 1375–1378.

63. World Health Organization. 2019. *Delivered by women, led by men: A gender and equity analysis of the global health and social workforce*. WHO.

64. Boniol, M., McIsaac, M., Xu, L., Wuliji, T., Diallo, K., and Campbell, J. 2019. *Gender equity in the health workforce: Analysis of 104 countries* (Working paper WHO/ HIS/HWF/Gender/WP1/2019.1). World Health Organization.

Chapter 3

1. Heggenhougen, H. K. 2009. Planting "seeds of health" in the fields of structural violence: The life and death of Francisco Curruchiche. In *Global health in times of violence*, 181–200, School for Advanced Research Press; Comisión para el Esclarecimiento Histórico (Guatemala). 2012. *Memory of silence: The Guatemalan truth commission report*.

2. Dinesen, C., Ronsbo, H., Juárez, C., González, M., Estrada Méndez, M.Á., and Modvig, J. 2013. Violence and social capital in post-conflict Guatemala. *Revista Panamericana de Salud Publica*, 34: 162–168; Flores, W., Ruano, A. L., and Funchal, D. P. 2009. Social participation within a context of political violence: Implications for the promotion and exercise of the right to health in Guatemala. *Health and Human Rights*, 11: 37; Abom, B. 2004. Social capital, NGOs, and development: A Guatemalan case study. *Development in Practice*, 14(3): 342–353.

3. Farmer, P. 2004. An anthropology of structural violence. *Current Anthropology*, 45(3): 305–325.

4. Green, L. 1999. *Fear as a way of life: Mayan widows in rural Guatemala*. Columbia University Press.

5. USAID. 2015. *Guatemala health assessment 2015*, accessed June 2, 2022, https://www.usaid.gov/sites/default/files/documents/1862/Guatemala-HSA%20_ENG-FULL-REPORT-FINAL-APRIL-2016.pdf.

6. Republica de Guatemala. 2014. *Encuesta Nacional de Condiciones de Vida 2014*, accessed June 2, 2022, https://www.ine.gob.gt/sistema/uploads/2016/02/03/bwc7f6t7asbei4wmuexonr0oscpshkyb.pdf.

7. Republica de Guatemala. 2014. *Encuesta Nacional de Condiciones de Vida 2014*, accessed June 2, 2022, https://www.ine.gob.gt/sistema/uploads/2016/02/03/bwc7f6t7asbei4wmuexonr0oscpshkyb.pdf; USAID. 2015. *Guatemala health assessment 2015*, accessed June 2, 2022, https://www.usaid.gov/sites/default/files/documents/1862/Guatemala-HSA%20_ENG-FULL-REPORT-FINAL-APRIL-2016.pdf.

8. Further staffing, opening hours, and services are available in enhanced health posts. For additional information and a health establishment search, see Republica de Guatemala. 2022. *Ministerio de Salud Pública y Asistencia Social*, accessed June 2, 2022, https://establecimientosdesalud.mspas.gob.gt/.

9. USAID. 2015. *Guatemala health assessment 2015*, accessed June 2, 2022, https://www.usaid.gov/sites/default/files/documents/1862/Guatemala-HSA%20_ENG-FULL-REPORT-FINAL-APRIL-2016.pdf.

10. USAID. 2015. *Guatemala health assessment 2015*, accessed June 2, 2022, https://www.usaid.gov/sites/default/files/documents/1862/Guatemala-HSA%20_ENG-FULL-REPORT-FINAL-APRIL-2016.pdf.

11. Maupin, J. 2011. Divergent models of community health workers in highland Guatemala. *Human Organization*, 70(1): 44–53.

12. During the extension of health coverage program from 1999 to 2016, a two-tier system of community health workers was created in the government system: (1) health facilitators who were trained to collect epidemiological data and deliver basic medicines and (2) health guardians who were trained to share health and hygiene messages in their communities and refer to care in the health system. Except where meaningful, I simplify the heterogeneity of these roles under the term community health worker.

13. Eder, K., and García Pú, M. M. 2003. *Modelo de la medicina indígena Maya en Guatemala: Investigación participativa en Sipacapa, San Marcos; San Martín Jilotepeque, Chimaltenango y San Juan Icoy, Huehuetenango*. Asociación de Servicios Comunitarios de Salud.

14. Hall-Clifford, R. A. 2009. *Oral rehydration therapy in highland Guatemala: Long-term impacts of public health intervention on the self* (Doctoral dissertation), Boston University.

15. USAID. 2015. *Guatemala health assessment 2015*, accessed June 2, 2022, https://www.usaid.gov/sites/default/files/documents/1862/Guatemala-HSA%20_ENG-FULL-REPORT-FINAL-APRIL-2016.pdf.

16. The maternity care unit was donated by the government of South Korea in building trade relationships in 2015.

17. Roche, S., and Hall-Clifford, R. 2015. Making surgical missions a joint operation: NGO experiences of visiting surgical teams and the formal health care system in Guatemala. *Global Public Health*, 10(10): 1201–1214.

18. Bourdieu, P. 2003. Symbolic violence. In *Beyond French Feminisms* Célestin, R., DalMolin, E. and De Courtivron, I., eds. 23–26. Palgrave Macmillan.

19. Granovsky-Larsen, S. 2019. *Dealing with peace: The Guatemalan campesino movement and the post-conflict neoliberal state*. University of Toronto Press; Benson, P., Fischer, E. F., and Thomas, K. 2008. Resocializing suffering: Neoliberalism, accusation, and the sociopolitical context of Guatemala's new violence. *Latin American Perspectives*, 35(5): 38–58; Maupin, J. N. 2008. Remaking the Guatemalan midwife: Health care reform and midwifery training programs in highland Guatemala. *Medical Anthropology*, 27(4): 353–382; Rohloff, P., Díaz, A., and Dasgupta, S. 2011. "Beyond development": A critical appraisal of the emergence of small health care non-governmental organizations in rural Guatemala. *Human Organization*, 70(4): 427–437.

20. Short, N. 2016. *The international politics of post-conflict reconstruction in Guatemala*. Springer.

21. Keshavjee, S. 2014. *Blind spot: How neoliberalism infiltrated global health*. University of California Press.

22. Maupin, J. N. 2009. "Fruit of the accords": Healthcare reform and civil participation in highland Guatemala. *Social Science & Medicine*, 68(8): 1456–1463.

23. Maupin, J. N. 2009. "Fruit of the accords": Healthcare reform and civil participation in highland Guatemala. *Social Science & Medicine*, 68(8): 1456–1463.

24. World Bank. 2013. *Improving access to health care services through the expansion of coverage program (PEC): The case of Guatemala*, accessed May 15, 2022, https://openknowledge.worldbank.org/bitstream/handle/10986/13283/75001.pdf?sequence=1&isAllowed=y.

25. World Bank. 2013. *Improving access to health care services through the expansion of coverage program (PEC): The case of Guatemala*, accessed May 15, 2022, https://openknowledge.worldbank.org/bitstream/handle/10986/13283/75001.pdf?sequence=1&isAllowed=y.

26. USAID. 2015. *Guatemala health assessment 2015*, accessed June 2, 2022, https://www.usaid.gov/sites/default/files/documents/1862/Guatemala-HSA%20_ENG-FULL-REPORT-FINAL-APRIL-2016.pdf.

27. USAID. 2015. *Guatemala health assessment 2015*, accessed June 2, 2022, https://www.usaid.gov/sites/default/files/documents/1862/Guatemala-HSA%20_ENG-FULL-REPORT-FINAL-APRIL-2016.pdf.

28. Pan American Health Organization (PAHO). 2007. *Health situation analysis and trends summary*, accessed October 2, 2017, https://www1.paho.org/english/gov/ce/od328-analysis-e.pdf

29. Rylko-Bauer, B., Whiteford, L. M., and Farmer, P. eds. 2009. Prologue. In *Global health in times of violence*, 3–16, School for Advanced Research Press.

30. The urban Chimaltenango health center is on the same grounds as the departmental hospital, so patients using this health center as their primary level of health care are more likely to be admitted as inpatients because of their proximity to the hospital.

31. The average is reduced to seven days when an outlier patient who reportedly had diarrhea for forty days before being brought to the government hospital is excluded.

32. Heggenhougen, H. K. 1976. *Health care for the "edge of the world": Indian campesinos as health workers in Chimaltenango, Guatemala. A discussion of the Behrhorst program* (Doctoral dissertation), Department of Anthropology, New School for Social Research.

33. Goldman, N., Pebley, A. R., and Gragnolati, M. 2002. Choices about treatment for ARI and diarrhea in rural Guatemala. *Social Science & Medicine*, 55: 1693–1712.

34. Adams, V. 2016. Introduction. In V. Adams (Ed.), *Metrics: What counts in global health*, 1–18, Duke University Press.

35. Nelson, D. M. 2015. *Who counts? The mathematics of death and life after genocide.* Duke University Press.

36. The NGO model further inscribes gender disparities by failures to acknowledge women's unpaid time and labor, often the basis of program implementation, and by positioning them as passive recipients to be "empowered" (Moore, J., Webb, M.F., Chary, A., Díaz, A.K. and Rohloff, P., 2017. Aid and gendered subjectivity in rural Guatemala. The Journal of Development Studies, 53(12), pp. 2164–2178).

37. Harvey, T. S. 2008. Where there is no patient: An anthropological treatment of a biomedical category. *Culture, Medicine, and Psychiatry*, 32(4): 577–606.

38. Pratt, B., and de Vries, J. 2018. Community engagement in global health research that advances health equity. *Bioethics*, 32(7): 454–463; Hernández, A. R., Hurtig, A. K., Dahlblom, K., and San Sebastián, M. 2014. More than a checklist: A realist evaluation of supervision of mid-level health workers in rural Guatemala. *BMC Health Services Research*, 14(1): 1–12.

39. Gobierno de Guatemala. 2012. *El plan del Pacto Hambre Cero*, accessed May 15, 2022, https://www.transparencia.gob.gt/wp-content/uploads/2017/07/INF-2012-002.pdf.

40. WFP. 2023. World Food Programme: Guatemala. https://www.wfp.org/countries /guatemala.

41. Heggenhougen, H. K. 1976. *Health care for the "edge of the world": Indian campesinos as health workers in Chimaltenango, Guatemala. A discussion of the Behrhorst program* (Doctoral dissertation), Department of Anthropology, New School for Social Research; Luecke, R. 1993. A new dawn with fingers to the world. In R. Luecke (Ed.), *A new dawn in Guatemala: Toward a worldwide health vision*. Waveland.

42. Fúnez-Flores, J. I. 2022. Decolonial and ontological challenges in social and anthropological theory. *Theory, Culture & Society*, 39(6): 21–41.

43. Nelson, D. M. 2015. *Who counts? The mathematics of death and life after genocide*. Duke University Press; Adams, V. 2016. *Metrics: What counts in global health*. Duke University Press.

44. Foucault, M. 1975. *Discipline and punish* (A. Sheridan, Trans.). Gallimard.

45. Petryna, A. 2004. Biological citizenship: The science and politics of Chernobyl-exposed populations. *Osiris*, 19: 250–265.

46. Turner, B. S. 1992. *Regulating bodies: Essays in medical sociology*. Routledge.

Chapter 4

1. Restall, M. 2004. *Seven myths of the Spanish conquest*. Oxford University Press.

2. Smith, P. H. 1992. The state and development in historical perspective. In A. Stepan (Ed.), *The Americas: New interpretative essays*. Oxford University Press.

3. Smith, P. H. 1992. The state and development in historical perspective. In A. Stepan (Ed.), *The Americas: New interpretative essays*. Oxford University Press.

4. Galeano, E. 1973. *Open veins of Latin America: Five centuries of the pillage of a continent*. Monthly Review Press.

5. Taylor, C. 1997. *Return of Guatemala's refugees: Reweaving the torn*. Temple University Press.

6. Smith, P. H. 1992. The state and development in historical perspective. In A. Stepan (Ed.), *The Americas: New interpretative essays*. Oxford University Press.

7. Galeano, E. 1973. *Open veins of Latin America: Five centuries of the pillage of a continent*. Monthly Review Press.

8. Loker, W. M. 1999. Grit in the prosperity machine: Globalization and the rural poor in Latin America. In Loker, W., ed., *Globalization and the rural poor in Latin America*, 9–40. Lynne Rienner.

9. Dos Santos, T. 1970. The structure of dependence. *The American Economic Review*, 60(2), 231–236

10. Dos Santos, T. 1970. The structure of dependence. *The American Economic Review*, 60(2).

11. Galeano, E. 1973. *Open veins of Latin America: Five centuries of the pillage of a continent*. Monthly Review Press.

12. Gunder Frank, A. 1986. The development of underdevelopment. In P. F. Klaren and T. J. Bossert (Eds.), *Promise of development: Theories of change in Latin America*. 111–123, Westview.

13. Lechner, N. 1998. The transformations of politics. In F. Aguero and J. Stark (Eds.), *Fault lines of democracy in post-transition Latin America*. North-South Center Press.

14. Lechner, N. 1998. The transformations of politics. In F. Aguero and J. Stark (Eds.), *Fault lines of democracy in post-transition Latin America*. North-South Center Press.

15. World Bank. 2022. *Guatemala country overview*, accessed June 10, 2022, https://www.worldbank.org/en/country/guatemala/overview.

16. World Bank. 2022. *Guatemala country overview*, accessed June 10, 2022, https://www.worldbank.org/en/country/guatemala/overview.

17. Inter-American Development Bank. 2022. *Guatemala: IDB country strategy, 2021–2024*, accessed June 10, 2022, https://idbdocs.iadb.org/wsdocs/getdocument.aspx?docnum=EZSHARE-1796625814-5.

18. Loker, W. M. 1999. Grit in the prosperity machine: Globalization and the rural poor in Latin America. In Loker, W. Ed., *Globalization and the rural poor in Latin America*, 9–40 Lynne Rienner; World Bank. 2022. *Guatemala country overview*, accessed June 10, 2022, https://www.worldbank.org/en/country/guatemala/overview.

19. World Bank. 2022. *Guatemala country overview*, accessed June 10, 2022, https://www.worldbank.org/en/country/guatemala/overview.

20. UNICEF. 2022. *Guatemala at a glance: Guatemala statistics*, accessed December 10, 2022, https://data.unicef.org/country/gtm/.

21. World Bank. 2022. *Guatemala country overview*, accessed June 10, 2022, https://www.worldbank.org/en/country/guatemala/overview.

22. World Bank. 2020. *Poverty and equity brief: Latin America and the Caribbean*, accessed June 10, 2022, https://databank.worldbank.org/data/download/poverty/33EF03BB-9722-4AE2-ABC7-AA2972D68AFE/Global_POVEQ_GTM.pdf; OECD. 2021. *Latin American economic outlook 2021: Working together for a better recovery*, accessed June 10, 2022, https://www.oecd-ilibrary.org/sites/633246fd-en/index.html?itemId=%2Fcontent%2Fcomponent%2F633246fd-en.

23. Fischer, E. F., and Benson, P. 2006. *Broccoli and desire: Global connections and maya struggles in postwar Guatemala*. Stanford University Press.

24. Nash, J. C. 2007. *Practicing ethnography in a globalizing world*. AltaMira Press.

25. Luecke, R. 1993. A new dawn with fingers to the world. In R. Luecke (Ed.), *A new dawn in Guatemala: Toward a worldwide health vision*. Waveland.

26. Behrhorst, C. 1983. Introduction. In U. Steltzer (Ed.), *Health in the Guatemalan Highlands*. University of Washington Press; Crawshaw, R. 1993. Human being and physician. In R. Luecke (Ed.), *A new dawn in Guatemala: Toward a worldwide health vision*. Waveland.

27. Behrhorst, C. 1983. Introduction. In U. Steltzer (Ed.), *Health in the Guatemalan Highlands*. University of Washington Press.

28. Luecke, R. 1993. A new dawn with fingers to the world. In R. Luecke (Ed.), *A new dawn in Guatemala: Toward a worldwide health vision*. Waveland.

29. Crawshaw, R. 1993. Human being and physician. In R. Luecke (Ed.), *A new dawn in Guatemala: Toward a worldwide health vision*. Waveland.

30. Luecke, R. 1993. A new dawn with fingers to the world. In R. Luecke (Ed.), *A new dawn in Guatemala: Toward a worldwide health vision*. Waveland.

31. Luecke, R. 1993. A new dawn with fingers to the world. In R. Luecke (Ed.), *A new dawn in Guatemala: Toward a worldwide health vision*. Waveland.

32. Luecke, R. 1993. A new dawn with fingers to the world. In R. Luecke (Ed.), *A new dawn in Guatemala: Toward a worldwide health vision*. Waveland.

33. Luecke, R. 1993. A new dawn with fingers to the world. In R. Luecke (Ed.), *A new dawn in Guatemala: Toward a worldwide health vision*. Waveland; Heggenhougen, H. K. 1976. *Health care for the "edge of the world": Indian campesinos as health workers in Chimaltenango, Guatemala. A discussion of the Behrhorst program* (Doctoral dissertation), Department of Anthropology, New School for Social Research.

34. Behrhorst, C. 1983. Introduction. In U. Steltzer (Ed.), *Health in the Guatemalan Highlands*. University of Washington Press.

35. Maupin, J. 2015. Strategic alliances: The shifting motivations for NGO collaboration with government programs. In A. Chary and P. Rohloff (Eds.), *Privatization and the new medical pluralism: Shifting healthcare landscapes in Maya Guatemala*, 3–18. Lexington Books.

36. Pellegrino, E. D. 1999. The commodification of medical and health care: the moral consequences of a paradigm shift from a professional to a market ethic. *Journal of Medicine and Philosophy*, 24(3): 243–266.

37. Hall-Clifford, A. R. 2009. *Oral rehydration therapy in highland Guatemala: Long-term impacts of public health intervention on the self* (Doctoral dissertation), Boston University.

38. Hueveline, P., and Noreen, G. 2000. A description of child illness and treatment behavior in Guatemala. *Social Science & Medicine*, 50: 345–364.

39. Pan American Health Organization (PAHO). 2007. *Health systems profile Guatemala*, accessed July 30, 2022, https://www.paho.org/hq/dmdocuments/2010/Health_System_Profile-Guatemala_2007.pdf.

40. Van der Geest, S. 1991. Marketplace conversations in Cameroon: How and why popular medical knowledge comes into being. *Culture, Medicine, and Psychiatry*, 15(1): 69–90.

41. Omnilife. 2022. *Centros de distribución*, accessed July 30, 2022, https://creoomnilife.zendesk.com/hc/es-419/categories/360002441632-Centros-de-distribuci%C3%B3n.

42. Cahn, P. S. 2006. Building down and dreaming up: Finding faith in a Mexican multilevel marketer. *American Ethnologist*, 33(1): 126–142; Sethi, R. 2014. A study of direct selling in India with special reference to Amway. *International Journal of Economics and Management*, 1(1): 43–55.

43. Hall-Clifford, R. 2015. Capitalizing on care: Marketplace quasi-pharmaceuticals in the Guatemalan health-seeking landscape. In A. Chary and P. Rohloff (Eds.), *Privatization and the new medical pluralism: Shifting healthcare landscapes in Maya Guatemala.*, 71–88 Lexington Books.

44. Akinladejo, O. H., Clarke, M., and Akinladejo, F. O. 2013. Pyramid schemes and multilevel marketing (MLM): Two sides of the same coin. *Journal of Modern Accounting and Auditing*, 9(5): 690–696.

45. Cahn, P. S. 2006. Building down and dreaming up: Finding faith in a Mexican multilevel marketer. *American Ethnologist*, 33(1): 126–142.

46. Hall-Clifford, R. 2015. Capitalizing on care: Marketplace quasi-pharmaceuticals in the Guatemalan health-seeking landscape. In A. Chary and P. Rohloff (Eds.), *Privatization and the new medical pluralism: Shifting healthcare landscapes in Maya Guatemala*. Lexington Books.

47. Omnilife and other similar quasi-pharmaceutical companies continue to be popular, though Omnilife's popularity seems to have peaked around 2015 in Guatemala.

48. Hall-Clifford, R. 2015. Capitalizing on care: Marketplace quasi-pharmaceuticals in the Guatemalan health-seeking landscape. In A. Chary and P. Rohloff (Eds.), *Privatization and the new medical pluralism: Shifting healthcare landscapes in Maya Guatemala*. Lexington Books.

49. Flood, D., and Rohloff, P. 2015. Diabetes in Indigenous Maya communities. In A. Chary and P. Rohloff (Eds.), *Privatization and the new medical pluralism: Shifting healthcare landscapes in Maya Guatemala*. Lexington Books.

50. Nelson, D. M. 2013. 100 percent Omnilife: Health, economy, and the end/s of war. In C. McAllister and D. M. Nelson (Eds.), *War by other means: Aftermath in postgenocide Guatemala*, 285–306. Duke University Press.

51. Fischer, E. F., and Benson, P. 2006. *Broccoli and desire: Global connections and Maya struggles in postwar Guatemala*. Stanford University Press; Goldin, L. R. 2011. *Global Maya: Work and ideology in rural Guatemala*. University of Arizona Press.

52. Nelson, D. M. 2013. 100 percent Omnilife: Health, economy, and the end/s of war. In C. McAllister and D. M. Nelson (Eds.), *War by other means: Aftermath in postgenocide Guatemala*, 285–306. Duke University Press.

53. Heggenhougen, H. K. 1976. *Health care for the "edge of the world": Indian campesinos as health workers in Chimaltenango, Guatemala. A discussion of the Behrhorst program* (Doctoral dissertation), Department of Anthropology, New School for Social Research.

54. I use the term "local healers" to acknowledge embeddedness in community culture, belief, traditions, and contemporary realities. The commonly used "traditional healers" implies an anachronism at odds with the dynamism of contemporary local healing practices. They are fully contemporary practitioners.

55. Hall-Clifford, R. A. 2009. *Oral rehydration therapy in highland Guatemala: Long-term impacts of public health intervention on the self* (Doctoral dissertation), Boston University.

56. Interestingly, this accords with Kendall et al.'s (1984) findings in Honduras that the population was open to ORT in all cases of diarrhea except those considered to be empacho, which local healers felt required a laxative to treat. Kendall, C., Foote, D., and Martorell, R. 1984. Ethnomedicine and oral rehydration therapy: A case study of ethnomedical investigation and program planning. *Social Science & Medicine*, 19: 253–260.

57. Hueveline, P., and Noreen, G. 2000. A description of child illness and treatment behavior in Guatemala. *Social Science & Medicine*, 50: 345–364; Eder, K., and García Pú, M. M. 2003. *Modelo de la medicina indígena Maya en Guatemala: Investigación participativa en Sipacapa, San Marcos; San Martín Jilotepeque, Chimaltenango y San Juan Ixcoy, Huehuetenango*. Asociación de Servicios Comunitarios de Salud.

58. Heggenhougen, H. K. 1976. *Health care for the "edge of the world": Indian campesinos as health workers in Chimaltenango, Guatemala. A discussion of the Behrhorst program* (Doctoral dissertation), Department of Anthropology, New School for Social Research.

59. Kawachi, I., and Berkman, L. 2000. Social cohesion, social capital, and health. In *Social Epidemiology*, 174–190, Oxford University Press.

60. Kenya, P.R., Gatiti S., Muthami L.N., Agwanda R., Mwenesi H.A., Katsivo M.N., et al. 1990. Oral rehydration therapy and social marketing in rural Kenya. *Social Science & Medicine*, 31(9): 979–987.

61. Van der Geest, S. 1991. Marketplace conversations in Cameroon: How and why popular medical knowledge comes into being. *Culture, Medicine, and Psychiatry*, 15(1): 69–90.

62. Van der Geest, S. 1991. Marketplace conversations in Cameroon: How and why popular medical knowledge comes into being. *Culture, Medicine, and Psychiatry*, 15(1): 69–90.

63. Black, R. E. 2001. Diarrheal diseases. In K. E. Nelson, C. M. Williams, and N. M. H. Graham (Eds.), *Infectious disease epidemiology: Theory and practice*. Aspen.

64. Gobierno de Guatemala. 2019. *Ministerio de Salud Pública y Asistencia Social Acuerdo ministerial número 181–2019*, accessed June 17, 2022, https://medicamentos .mspas.gob.gt/index.php/legislacion-vigente/acuerdos?download=300%3Apara-la -regulacion-de-medicamentos-de-prescripcion-medica-antimicrobianos-y-esteroides -oftalmicos-version-2.

65. Martiniuk A. L., Manouchehrian, M., Negin, J. A., and Zwi, A. B. 2012. Brain gains: A literature review of medical missions to low and middle-income countries. *BMC Health Services Research*, 12(1): 134; Sykes K. J. 2014. Short-term medical service trips: A systematic review of the evidence. *American Journal of Public Health*, 104(7): 38–48.

66. Roche, S., Brockington, M., Fathima, S., Nandi, M., Silverberg, B., Rice, H. E., and Hall-Clifford, R. 2018. Freedom of choice, expressions of gratitude: Patient experiences of short-term surgical missions in Guatemala. *Social Science & Medicine*, 208(2018): 117–125.

67. Roche, S., and Hall-Clifford, R. 2015. Making surgical missions a joint operation: NGO experiences of visiting surgical teams and the formal health care system in Guatemala. *Global Public Health*, 10(10): 1201–1214.

68. Roche, S., Brockington, M., Fathima, S., Nandi, M., Silverberg, B., Rice, H. E., and Hall-Clifford, R. 2018. Freedom of choice, expressions of gratitude: Patient experiences of short-term surgical missions in Guatemala. *Social Science & Medicine*, 208(2018): 117–125.

69. Berry, N. S. 2014. Did we do good? NGOs, conflicts of interest and the evaluation of short-term medical missions in Sololá, Guatemala. *Social Science & Medicine*, 120 (2014): 344–351; Lasker, J. N. 2015. *Hoping to help*. Cornell University Press; Sullivan, N. 2018. International clinical volunteering in Tanzania: A postcolonial analysis of a Global Health business. *Global Public Health*, 13(3): 310–324; Sullivan, N., and Berry, N. 2017. Good intentions and murky ethics. *Anthropology News*, 58(6): e61–e67.

70. Roche, S., Brockington, M., Fathima, S., Nandi, M., Silverberg, B., Rice, H. E., and Hall-Clifford, R. 2018. Freedom of choice, expressions of gratitude: Patient experiences of short-term surgical missions in Guatemala. *Social Science & Medicine*, 208(2018): 117–125.

71. Colegio De Médicos y Cirujanos De Guatemala. 2017. Inscripción de medicos extranjeros. https://colmedegua.org/web/wp-content/uploads/2017/03/INSTRUCTIVO _JOR_MED.pdf.

72. Nouvet, E. 2016. Extra-ordinary aid and its shadows: The work of gratitude in Nicaraguan humanitarian healthcare. *Critique of Anthropology*, 36(3): 244–263.

73. Roche, S., Brockington, M., Fathima, S., Nandi, M., Silverberg, B., Rice, H. E., and Hall-Clifford, R. 2018. Freedom of choice, expressions of gratitude: Patient experiences of short-term surgical missions in Guatemala. *Social Science & Medicine*, 208(2018): 117–125.

74. Roche, S. and Rachel Hall-Clifford, R. 2015. Making surgical missions a joint operation: NGO experiences of visiting surgical teams and the formal health care system in Guatemala. *Global Public Health*, 10(10): 1201–1214.

75. Chary, A., Messmer, S., Sorenson, E., Henretty, N., Dasgupta, S., and Rohloff, P. 2013. The normalization of childhood disease: An ethnographic study of child malnutrition in rural Guatemala. *Human Organization*, 72(2): 87–97; Rohloff, P. 2021. On the frontlines of chronic paediatric undernutrition in Guatemala. *eBioMedicine*, 64: 103223; Coarasa, J., Das, J., Gummerson, E., and Bitton, A. 2017. A systematic tale of two differing reviews: Evaluating the evidence on public and private sector quality of primary care in low and middle income countries. *Globalization and Health*, 13(1): 1–7; Zielinski Gutiérrez, E. C., and Kendall, C. 2000. The globalization of health and disease: The health transition and global change. In G. L. Albrecht, R. Fitzpatrick, and S. C. Scrimshaw (Eds.), *Handbook of Social Studies in Health and Medicine*. Sage.

76. Keshavjee, S. 2014. *Blind spot: How neoliberalism infiltrated global health*. University of California Press.

77. Singer, M. 2008. *Drugs and development: The global impact on sustainable growth and human rights*. Waveland.

78. Cowen, D. 2014. *The deadly life of logistics: Mapping violence in global trade*. University of Minnesota Press.

79. Hannerz, U. 1992. *Cultural complexity: Studies in the social organization of meaning*. Columbia University Press.

80. Bourdieu, P. 2005. *The forms of capital*. Routledge.

Chapter 5

1. This colleague asked to remain anonymous.

2. Bornstein, E., and Redfield P. 2011. *Forces of compassion: Humanitarianism between ethics and politics*. SAR Press.

3. Keshavjee, S. 2014. *Blind spot: How neoliberalism infiltrated global health.* University of California Press.

4. Malkki, L. H. 2015. *The need to help: The domestic arts of international humanitarianism.* Duke University Press.

5. Han, C. 2014. The difficulty of kindness: Boundaries, time, and the ordinary. In V. Das, M. D. Jackson, A. Kleinman, and B. Singh (Eds.), *The ground between: Anthropologists engage philosophy*, 71–93. Duke University Press.

6. Feldman, I., and Miriam T. 2010. Introduction government and humanity. In *In the Name of Humanity*, 1–26. Duke University Press; Fassin, D. 2011. *Humanitarian reason: A moral history of the present.* University of California Press.

7. Benatar, S. R. 2013. Global health and justice: Re-examining our values. *Bioethics*, 27(7): 297–304.

8. Wilkinson, I., and Arthur K. 2016. *A passion for society: How we think about human suffering.* University of California Press.

9. Wallerstein, I. 1987. World-systems analysis. *Social Theory Today* 3.

10. Easterly, W. 2006. The white man's burden. *The Lancet*, 367(9528): 2060.

11. Packard, R. M. 2016. *A history of global health: Interventions into the lives of other peoples.* Johns Hopkins University Press.

12. Brown, P. J. 2016. The four 19th century roots of international and global health: A model for understanding current policy debates. In P. J. Brown and S. Closser (Eds.), Foundations of Global Health: An Interdisciplinary Reader, 344–354, Oxford.

13. Brown, P. J. 2016. The four 19th century roots of international and global health: A model for understanding current policy debates. In P. J. Brown and S. Closser (Eds.), *Foundations of Global Health: An Interdisciplinary Reader*, 344–354 Oxford; Van der Geest, S., Speckmann, J. D., and Streefland, P. H. 1990. Primary health care in a multi-level perspective: Towards a research agenda. *Social Science & Medicine*, 30(9): 1025–1034.

14. Abel, C. and Lloyd-Sherlock P. 2000. Health policy in Latin America: Themes, trends and challenges. In Lloyd-Sherlock P. (Ed.), *Healthcare reform and poverty in Latin America.* Institute of Latin American Studies.

15. Schoultz, L. 1981. *Human rights and United States policy toward Latin America.* Princeton University Press; Keck, M. E., and Sikkink K. 1998. *Activists beyond borders: Advocacy networks in international politics.* Cornell University Press.

16. Risse, T., and Sikkink K. 1999. The socialization of international human rights norms into domestic practices: Introduction. In T. Risse, S. C. Ropp, and K. Sikkink

(Eds.), *The power of human rights: International norms and domestic change*. Cambridge: Cambridge University Press.

17. Risse, T., and Sikkink K. 1999. The socialization of international human rights norms into domestic practices: Introduction. In T. Risse, S. C. Ropp, and K. Sikkink (Eds.), *The power of human rights: International norms and domestic change*. Cambridge: Cambridge University Press.

18. Keck, M. E., and Sikkink K. 1998. *Activists beyond borders: Advocacy networks in international politics*. Cornell University Press; Cogburn, D. L. 2017. *Transnational advocacy networks in the information society: Partners or pawns?* Springer.

19. Heggenhougen, H. K. 1984. Will primary health care efforts be allowed to succeed? *Social Science & Medicine* 19(3): 217–224; van der Geest, S., Speckmann, J. D. and Streefland, P. H. 1990. Primary health care in a multi-level perspective: Towards a research agenda. *Social Science & Medicine* 30(9): 1025–1034.

20. Farmer, P. 2004b. *Pathologies of power: Health, human rights, and the new war on the poor*. University of California Press.

21. United Nations. *Millennium Development Goals*, accessed July 31, 2022, https://research.un.org/en/docs/dev/2000-2015#:~:text=Introduction%2C%202000%2D2015&text=The%20Millennium%20Development%20Goals%20set,Eradicate%20extreme%20poverty%20and%20hunger.

22. McCoy, D., and Linsey M. 2011. Global health and the Gates Foundation—in perspective. In *Partnerships and foundations in global health governance*, 143–163. Palgrave Macmillan; Fergus, C. A. 2022. Power across the global health landscape: A network analysis of development assistance 1990–2015. *Health Policy and Planning*, 37(6): 779–790.

23. Adams, V. 2016. *Metrics: What counts in global health*. Duke University Press.

24. World Health Organization. 2021. *Universal health coverage (UCH)*, accessed July 22, 2022, https://www.who.int/news-room/fact-sheets/detail/universal-health-coverage-(uhc).

25. Sachs, J. D. 2012. From millennium development goals to sustainable development goals. *The Lancet*, 379(9832): 2206–2211.

26. Adams, V. 2016. *Metrics: What counts in global health*. Duke University Press.

27. I am part of this bureaucracy because of the privileges of my birth, training, and employment in high-income country contexts as a dual US/UK citizen. See the pressure points for action and change at the end of this chapter and my reflections in the conclusion of this book for further discussion.

28. Easterly, W. 2014. *The tyranny of experts: Economists, dictators, and the forgotten rights of the poor*. Basic Books.

29. The poverty level is defined as living on US$1.90 per day or less.

30. World Health Organization. 2021. *Universal health coverage (UCH)*, accessed July 22, 2022, https://www.who.int/news-room/fact-sheets/detail/universal-health -coverage-(uhc).

31. World Bank. 2017. *Tracking universal health coverage: 2017 global monitoring report*, accessed July 22, 2022, https://www.worldbank.org/en/topic/universalhealth coverage/publication/tracking-universal-health-coverage-2017-global-monitoring -report.

32. Congressional Research Service. 2022. *Foreign assistance: An Introduction to U.S. programs and policy 2022*, accessed July 22, 2022, https://sgp.fas.org/crs/row/R40213 .pdf.

33. Abel, C., and Lloyd-Sherlock P. 2000. Health policy in Latin America: Themes, trends and challenges. In Lloyd-Sherlock P. (Ed.), *Healthcare reform and poverty in Latin America*. Institute of Latin American Studies.

34. Abel, C. and Lloyd-Sherlock P. 2000. Health policy in Latin America: Themes, trends and challenges. In Lloyd-Sherlock P. (Ed.), *Healthcare reform and poverty in Latin America*. Institute of Latin American Studies.

35. Pan American Health Organization (PAHO). 2017. *PAHO program and budget 2018–2019*, accessed August 11, 2022, https://iris.paho.org/handle/10665.2/34467.

36. Rohloff, P., Diaz, A. K., and Dasgupta S. 2011. Beyond development: A critical appraisal of the emergence of small health care non-governmental organizations in rural Guatemala. *Human Organization*, 70(4): 427–437.

37. Douglas, M. 1973. *Natural symbols: Explorations in cosmology*. Routledge.

38. Foucault, M. 1973. *The birth of the clinic: An archaeology of medical perception*. A.M. Sheridan, trans. Tavistock; Turner, B. 1992. *Regulating bodies: Essays in medical sociology*. Routledge.

39. Outcry over misdirected funding allocated for the COVID-19 pandemic response is representative of the kinds of systemic seepage from the government health system coffers that citizens have come to expect (Prensa Comunitaria. 2021. *Guatemala, la crisis de las vacunas y la corrupción*, accessed June 1, 2023, https://www.prensacomunitaria .org/2021/07/guatemala-la-crisis-de-las-vacunas-y-la-corrupcion/).

40. Singer, P. 2015. What is effective altruism? In *The most good you can do*, 3–12. Yale University Press.

41. World Bank. 2018. *Guatemala's water supply, sanitation, and hygiene poverty diagnostic: Challenges and opportunities*. International Bank for Reconstruction and Development/World Bank. https://openknowledge.worldbank.org/bitstream/handle /10986/29454/W17026.pdf?sequence=7.

42. Ranabhat, C. L., Mihajlo J., Meghnath D. and Kim C.-B. 2020. Structural factors responsible for universal health coverage in low-and middle-income countries: Results from 118 countries. *Frontiers in Public Health* 7: 414.

43. Marmot, M. 2005. Social determinants of health inequalities. *The Lancet*, 365: 1099–1104.

44. Fischer, E. F. 1996. Induced culture change as a strategy for socioeconomic development: The pan-Maya movement in Guatemala. In E. F. Fischer and R. McKenna Brown (Eds.), *Maya Cultural Activism in Guatemala*, 51–73, University of Texas Press; Brysk, A. 2000. *From tribal village to global village: Indian rights and international relations in Latin America*. Stanford University Press.

45. Jackson, J.E., and Warren, K.B. 2005. "Indigenous Movements in Latin America, 1992–2004: Controversies, Ironies, New Directions." Annual Review of Anthropology 34: 549–573.

46. Farmer, P. 2004. An anthropology of structural violence. *Current Anthropology*, 45(3): 305–325.

47. Polgar, S. 1962. Health and human behavior: Areas of interest common to the social and medical sciences. *Current Anthropology*, 3(2): 159–205.

48. Guttman, N., and Ressler, W. H. 2001. On being responsible: Ethical issues in appeals to personal responsibility in health campaigns. *Journal of Health Communication*, 6: 117–136.

49. Guttman, N., and Ressler, W. H. 2001. On being responsible: Ethical issues in appeals to personal responsibility in health campaigns. *Journal of Health Communication*, 6: 117–136.

50. Wayland, C., and Crowder, J. 2002. Disparate views of community in primary health care: Understanding how perceptions influence success. *Medical Anthropology Quarterly*, 16(2): 230–247.

51. Lavery, J. V. 2018. Building an evidence base for stakeholder engagement. *Science*, 361(6402): 554–556.

52. Woelk, G. B. 1992. Cultural and structural influences in the creation of and participation in community health programmes. *Social Science & Medicine*, 35(4): 419–424.

53. World Health Organization. 2019. *Delivered by women, led by men: A gender and equity analysis of the global health and social workforce*. WHO.

54. Flores, W., and Gómez-Sánchez, I. 2010. La gobernanza en los Consejos Municipales de Desarrollo de Guatemala: Análisis de actores y relaciones de poder. *Revista de Salud Pública*, 12: 138–150.

55. Galtung, J. 1990. Cultural violence. *Journal of Peace Research*, 27(3): 291–305.

56. Prüss-Üstün, A. and C. Corvalán. 2007. *Preventing disease through healthy environments: Towards an estimate of the environmental burden of disease*. WHO. https://www.who.int/publications/i/item/9789241565196; Eder, K., and García Pú, M. M. 2003. *Modelo de la medicina indígena Maya en Guatemala: Investigación participativa en Sipacapa, San Marcos; San Martín Jilotepeque, Chimaltenango y San Juan Ixcoy, Huehuetenango*. Asociación de Servicios Comunitarios de Salud.

57. Chiller, T. M., Mendoza, C. E., Beatriz Lopez, M., Alvarez, M., Hoekstra, R. M., Keswick, B. H., and Luby, S. P. 2006. Reducing diarrhoea in Guatemalan children: Randomized controlled trial of flocculant-disinfectant for drinking-water. *Bulletin of the World Health Organization*, 84(1): 28–35.

58. Pellmar, T. C., Brandt, E. N., Jr., and Baird M. A. 2002. Health and behavior: The interplay of biological, behavioral, and social influences: Summary of an Institute of Medicine Report. *American Journal of Health Promotion*, 16(4): 206–219; Ruano, A. L., Sánchez S., Jerez, F. J., and Flores, W. 2014. Making the post-MDG global health goals relevant for highly inequitable societies: Findings from a consultation with marginalized populations in Guatemala. *International Journal for Equity in Health*, 13(1): 1–8.

59. Werner, D., and Sanders, D. 1997. *Questioning the solution: The politics of primary care and child survival*. HealthWrights. Werner, D., Sanders, D., and Weston, J. 1997. *Questioning the solution: The politics of primary health care and child survival, with an in-depth critique of oral rehydration therapy*.

60. Ferguson, J. 1994. *The anti-politics machine: "Development," depoliticization, and bureaucratic power in Lesotho*. University of Minnesota Press.

61. Schuller, M. 2012. *Killing with kindness: Haiti, international aid, and NGOs*. Rutgers University Press.

62. Benton, A. 2015. *HIV exceptionalism: Development through disease in Sierra Leone*. University of Minnesota Press.

63. Binagwaho, A., Farmer, P. E., Nsanzimana, S., Karema, C., Gasana, M., de Dieu Ngirabega, J., Ngabo, F., et al. 2014. "Rwanda 20 years on: Investing in life." *The Lancet*, 384(9940): 371–375.

64. Ferguson, J. 1994. *The anti-politics machine: "Development," depoliticization, and bureaucratic power in Lesotho*. University of Minnesota Press.

65. Sheel, M., and Martyn D. K. 2018. Parasitic and parachute research in global health. *The Lancet Global Health*, 6(8): e839; Naidu, T. 2021. Says who? Northern ventriloquism, or epistemic disobedience in global health scholarship. *The Lancet Global Health*, 9(9): e1332–e1335; Sayeed, S., and Taylor L. 2020. Institutionalising global health: A call for ethical reflection. *BMJ Global Health*, 5(9): e003353.

66. Abimbola, Seye, Sumegha Asthana, Cristian Montenegro, Renzo R. Guinto, Desmond Tanko Jumbam, Lance Louskieter, Kenneth Munge Kabubei et al. "Addressing power asymmetries in global health: imperatives in the wake of the COVID-19 pandemic." PLoS medicine 18, no. 4 (2021): e1003604.

67. Prasad, S., Aldrink, M., Compton, B., Lasker, J., Donkor, P., Weakliam, D., Rowthorn, V., et al. 2022. Global health partnerships and the Brocher declaration: Principles for ethical short-term engagements in global health. *Annals of Global Health*, 88(1).

68. Figueredo, A., and Chowdhury, R. 2019. Conceptualization of community-based entrepreneurship: A case study of Ecofiltro in Guatemala. *European Association of Work and Organizational Psychology in Practice*, 2(11): 77–101.

69. Richardson, E., Phillips, M., Colom, A., Khalil, I., and Nichols, J. 2019. Out of school factors affecting Indigenous girls' educational attainment: A theory of change for the opening opportunities program in rural Guatemala. *Comparative and International Education*, 47(2); Hernández, A., Hurtig, A.-K., Goicolea, I., Sebastián, M. S., Jerez, F., Hernández-Rodríguez, F., and Flores, W. 2020. Building collective power in citizen-led initiatives for health accountability in Guatemala: The role of networks. *BMC Health Services Research*, 20(1): 1–14.

Conclusion

1. Roth, G. A., Abate, D., Abate, K. H., Abay, S. M., Abbafati, C., Abbasi, N., Abbastabar, H., et al. 2018. Global, regional, and national age-sex-specific mortality for 282 causes of death in 195 countries and territories, 1980–2017: A systematic analysis for the Global Burden of Disease Study 2017. *The Lancet*, 392(10159): 1736–1788.

2. Hall-Clifford, R., and Cook-Deegan, R. 2019. Ethically managing risks in global health fieldwork: Human rights ideals confront real world challenges. *Health and Human Rights*, 21(1): 7.

3. Hall-Clifford, R. 2020. Applied anthropology, activism, and loss: Experiences from highland Guatemala. *Annals of Anthropological Practice*, 44(2): 198–201.

4. Brown, P. J., and Closser, S. 2016. *Understanding and applying medical anthropology.* Routledge.

5. Holeman, I., and Kane, D. 2020. Human-centered design for global health equity. *Information Technology for Development*, 26(3): 477–505; Bazzano, A. N., Martin, J., Hicks, E., Faughnan, M., and Murphy, L. 2017. Human-centred design in global health: A scoping review of applications and contexts. *PLoS One*, 12(11): e0186744.

6. Bang, A. 2018. *Research, for whom.* India Development Review; Pratt, B., and de Vries, J. 2018. Community engagement in global health research that advances health equity. *Bioethics*, 32(7): 454–463.

7. Holeman, I., and Kane, D. 2020. Human-centered design for global health equity. *Information Technology for Development*, 26(3): 477–505.

8. Slattery, P., Saeri, A. K., and Bragge, P. 2020. Research co-design in health: A rapid overview of reviews. *Health Research Policy and Systems*, 18(1): 1–13.

9. Farr, M. 2018. Power dynamics and collaborative mechanisms in co-production and co-design processes. *Critical Social Policy*, 38(4): 623–644; Donetto, S., Pierri, P., Tsianakas, V., and Robert, G. 2015. Experience-based co-design and healthcare improvement: Realizing participatory design in the public sector. *The Design Journal*, 18(2): 227–248.

10. Charani, E., Abimbola, S., Pai, M., Adeyi, O., Mendelson, M., Laxminarayan, R., and Rasheed, M. A. 2022. Funders: The missing link in equitable global health research? *PLoS Global Public Health*, 2(6): e0000583.

11. Opara, I. N. 2021. It's time to decolonize the decolonization movement. *Speaking of Medicine and Health*, 29; Büyüm, A. M., Kenney, C., Koris, A., Mkumba, L., and Raveendran, Y. 2020. Decolonising global health: If not now, when? *BMJ Global Health*, 5(8): e003394.

Index